Penguin Health

# A GOOD START
## Healthy Eating in the First Five Years

Louise Graham was educated at London University. Her first degree was in physiology. She then studied at the Institute of Obstetrics and Gynaecology and obtained a PhD in clinical pharmacology. Subsequently, she was awarded a post-doctoral fellowship at the Royal Postgraduate Medical School, Hammersmith Hospital. She has contributed papers on neonatal jaundice to, among others, the *British Medical Journal*, the *Lancet* and the *British Journal of Clinical Pharmacology*.

She has previously written medical film scripts and held private classes in preparation for childbirth. She enjoys painting and lives in London with her husband and three young sons.

# A GOOD START
## HEALTHY EATING IN THE FIRST FIVE YEARS

**Louise Graham**

**Penguin Books**

Penguin Books Ltd, Harmondsworth, Middlesex, England
Viking Penguin Inc., 40 West 23rd Street, New York, New York 10010, U.S.A.
Penguin Books Australia Ltd, Ringwood, Victoria, Australia
Penguin Books Canada Limited, 2801 John Street, Markham, Ontario,
Canada L3R 1B4
Penguin Books (N.Z.) Ltd, 182–190 Wairau Road, Auckland 10, New Zealand

First published 1986

Filmset in Trump (Linotron 202) by
Rowland Phototypesetting Limited,
Bury St Edmunds, Suffolk
Made and printed in Great Britain by
Hazell Watson & Viney Limited,
Member of the BPCC Group
Aylesbury, Bucks

**FOR RICHARD**

# CONTENTS

# ACKNOWLEDGEMENTS

I am grateful to Rosemary Friedman for her literary help, Richard Graham for his constructive criticism and encouragement, and Camilla Straghan for her practical assistance in the preparation of the manuscript. I am also indebted to Dr Dennis Friedman for his medical and psychological advice relating to development in the first five years, and to my two sons Henry and Jack Graham who were willing guinea-pigs.

# INTRODUCTION

The constant poor health of a child eating an inferior diet is an enormous drain on parents, physically, psychologically and economically. Yet in our society, preventative medicine, in terms of taking responsibility for one's own or one's children's good health, is not rated sufficiently highly. Perhaps this is because many parents wrongly believe that they can do little to influence their child's health or appearance, or because they prefer to leave things to chance and seek help only when illness strikes.

The advertising pressures of the food-processing industry are constantly brought to bear on the family, while informed advice about what is healthiest is scarce and is often hard to interpret. I hope this book will help to redress the balance for those who care for young children. I believe that most parents are prepared to do their utmost for the well-being of their children, but are often unaware of how best to protect them from bad health, both in the short term and in later life.

This book illustrates not only why a diet of relatively unprocessed wholefoods is best for young children, but how such a regime can be followed simply and inexpensively. The first part explains the nutritional facts and theory, the second shows how to put it into practice.

Many parents may not be able to follow the 'ideal' diet to the letter, yet should at least know what to aim at and should understand why children should limit their consumption of highly refined foods, sugar, salt, white flour, artificial additives, certain fats and oils, and so on, but eat plenty of fresh produce rich in essential nutrients and dietary fibre.

Superior ingredients do not in themselves necessarily produce a good diet. The selection and preparation of a child's food is crucial in order to maximize nutritional value.

Optimum health through good nutrition is, I believe, one of the most important gifts that all parents can bestow on their children in the early years, and the benefits will last for their lifetime. These recommendations, which are based on my experiences with my own young family, will help all parents to give their children the best possible start.

# 1

# THE IMPORTANCE OF A GOOD DIET

Many of today's diseases are now known to be food-related. These 'Western' diseases, which often start their development during childhood but may not manifest themselves until adulthood, include high blood pressure, blood vessel and heart disease, tooth decay, constipation, diabetes, obesity, certain cancers and some cases of arthritis. Because of their exposure to junk foods, and their lower body weight, children are more vulnerable to disease caused by wrong eating than adults. A child's future health therefore depends on the way he is fed, particularly during the first few years.

A healthy diet from birth, based on unrefined foods and avoiding excess sugar, salt and fat, will be the child's best endowment, and the resulting health and vigour will stand him in good stead for the rest of his life. Strong bones, firm muscles, glowing skin, normal endocrine glands, a healthy liver, optimum reproductive capacity, superior intelligence and attractive appearance are as dependent upon correct diet as upon genetic make-up. Nourishing food need not be expensive. In those areas of the Third World where food supplies are adequate, a subsistence diet of vegetables and hard wholemeal bread or rice, with occasional small portions of meat or fish, maintains good health and extremely sound teeth.

Prior to the Second World War, when the science of nutrition was in its infancy, the average person had little knowledge of which foods were needed to establish or maintain good health. Many families were either not getting enough to eat, or consuming insufficient nutrients for proper growth. Deficiency diseases were common, and stunted growth, rickets, infectious illnesses and colds were endemic amongst children.

The balanced diet imposed by food rationing during the war resulted in a nation healthier than it has been at any time since. The incidence of infant mortality and anaemia fell and dental health and growth rates improved. After the war, as a result of expansion in the food-processing industry, new and different types of food became available and eating habits changed. Family meals became less common and the trend shifted from buying fresh produce towards convenience foods.

When the health of children (from birth to four years) born in 1946 was compared with that of their offspring, an increase in the prevalence of many illnesses requiring hospitalization was observed. The chances of admission to hospital in the first generation were 139 per thousand children as against 199 per thousand in the second generation. Other studies of children in this age group have shown a sixfold increase in eczema and childhood diabetes since 1946, a threefold increase in asthma, and a doubling in obesity.

## WHAT IS WRONG WITH EATING REFINED FOODS?

With the advances in food processing, more and more of the world's population abandoned its traditional diet of locally grown foods for the 'new' refined foods, and scientists took the opportunity of studying the effects that this switching of diet had on health. One such study demonstrated the devastating effect that refined foods can have on a previously healthy people. It was found that when primitive peoples ate their native foods, their facial bones were broad, their eyes widely spaced, their cheekbones well developed, and their jawbones sufficiently large to permit the teeth to be even and straight without overcrowding. Some people in these groups, who had adopted the worst features of a Western diet – chiefly foods which can be shipped without spoiling, such as canned foods, white flour products, refined sugar and coffee – showed dental caries, deformities in the facial bones and crowded mouths, previously unknown in their society. These malformations of the bones of the face and head were associated with lower IQs, personality disturbances and a dramatically higher incidence of the diseases commonly found in Western societies such as heart disease, diabetes and obesity.

Adults often eat a healthier diet than children, as the taste for sweets, desserts, soft drinks and sweet foods in general decreases with age. Parents will select meals consisting of plain grilled meat or fish, fresh vegetables and fruit for themselves, yet surprisingly buy fish-fingers, ready-made hamburgers, sausages, crisps, chips, instant gelatine desserts, artificial fruit drinks and other trash foods for their children, in the mistaken belief that they are 'more suitable'. It is sometimes difficult to resist the pressures of advertising and to forgo the saving in time and effort that these convenience foods offer to busy mothers. The importance of avoiding these processed foods cannot be overstated, however.

## SUGAR – THE WHITE PERIL

Crystalline table sugar is one of the purest chemicals regularly produced in large quantities by modern industry – 38kg (84 lb) per person are eaten each year. It is practically one hundred per cent sucrose and contains no essential nutrients. The body does not need sugar, since all nutritional requirements can be fulfilled without having to take a single spoon of sugar, on its own or in any food or drink. Medical evidence has indicted sugar as a major cause of diabetes, obesity, heart disease and tooth decay.

Sugar acts as an anti-nutrient – vitamins and minerals are required to metabolize the sugar, so a child eating a lot of it needs more vitamins, etc., in the rest of his diet than one who eats no sugar; in fact, he is likely to fill himself up on the sugar and to have less room for nutritive food.

The child's struggle against sugar and its associated health problems frequently begins at birth. Sugar water (dextrose) is offered to babies as a substitute for formula or colostrum (early breast milk) to enable mothers to adhere to fixed feeding schedules or get a night's sleep. Sugar water may harm the pancreas by stimulating the outflow of insulin too early in life. Sugar water and some infant formulas which are sweetened with sucrose or glucose encourage babies to develop a taste for refined sugar.

After weaning, most babies progress to sugary, vitamin-supplemented fruit syrups, rusks and commercial baby foods, and then on to sweetened children's breakfast cereals, jams, canned foods, sweets and biscuits, and a variety of highly processed foods containing sugar.

Obesity is probably the most common nutritional disorder associated with over-consumption of sugar, and fat children often become fat adults. Overweight children are especially prone to diabetes, heart disease, blood-vessel disease and many other diseases. Viruses, bacteria and fungi thrive on sweet skin, and some skin infections result from eating sugar. Recent research has suggested that behavioural disturbances, such as a hyperactivity, may also sometimes result from over-consumption of sugar.

## IS FAT OK?

The controversy continues to rage about the health risks and benefits of the various fats and oils that form a large part of the modern diet. What is least controversial is that any over-consumption of food – and fat is a concentrated source of energy – increases blood fats, and high levels of circulating fat are known to be associated with heart disease and other related conditions.

Babies need fat as an important source of energy and of fat-soluble vitamins, and it is also required by the rapidly growing brain and nerves. Breast milk, but not infant formulas, contains the ideal types and quantity of fat that babies need for optimum health. The fat content varies throughout the day, the amount being least in the early hours of the morning. There is a variation within any one feed, the 'hind' milk being richer in fat than the 'fore' milk. The fat in breast milk is also absorbed better than the fat in infant formulas.

After weaning, small amounts of certain essential fats are needed for maintaining good health and resistance to disease, and many vitamins (A, D, E and K) cannot be absorbed without fat. Problems occur, however, when too much fat, the wrong types of fat or stale fats are eaten. A child could easily be having too much fat in his diet if he regularly eats fried food or highly processed foods. All fats, whether they come from animal or vegetable sources, are potentially harmful to health when eaten in large quantities.

Animal fats – butter, cheese, cream, fat in meat, etc. – are highly saturated and although their consumption is linked to the development of heart disease, blood-vessel disease, strokes and certain cancers, they may well turn out to be preferable to many new oils – mainly expressed from vegetable seeds – which have not been around long enough for their long-term effects to be known. There are many primitive peoples, of widely differing ethnic stocks, who have always eaten a great deal of animal fat but who do not suffer from heart or artery disease to any significant extent. It is clear, therefore, that it is the total nutrition available to the body that matters in arterial health, rather than any one particular risk factor.

Potentially more harmful than either animal fats or pure vegetable oils are the hydrogenated fats found in margarine, refined salted oils, snack foods and commercial fried foods (fish and chips). These fats have been chemically modified to improve their keeping qualities. Hydrogenated fats have been shown to be related to deaths from blood-vessel disease.

Fats should always be eaten as fresh as possible – this is particularly true for vegetable oils – since rancid fats are damaging to health. Oil that has been heated for frying should not be re-used. Vegetable oils should be stored in a cool dark place. It should be remembered that most manufactured foods contain fats, and the staler these are, the more harmful they become.

## FIBRE – WHY IT IS NEEDED

Dietary fibre consists of those parts of leaves, stems, roots, seeds and fruits of plants that are not digested by enzymes produced in the human digestive system. It is not one substance, but a complex mixture of many different substances. Food sources of fibre are cereals, pulses, root vegetables and some leafy vegetables, nuts and fruits. Food processing often results in the removal of most, if not all of this fibre. White flour, for example, is almost totally lacking in dietary fibre (the bran), and when vegetables are peeled much of it is discarded. Fibre increases the bulk of the daily bowel motion, and lack of it in the diet has been held responsible for such commonplace Western diseases as constipation, coronary heart disease, cancer, gallstones, appendicitis, diabetes, obesity, haemorrhoids and varicose veins.

Most commercial baby foods contain very little fibre – cereals are usually refined and fruit and vegetables peeled – and for this reason alone they are best avoided. Few breakfast cereals are made from the whole grain and many that are contain added sugar and salt. A few high-fibre, sugar-free cereals have recently become available in response to public demand and medical opinion. A child who eats wholegrain bread and pasta, brown rice, etc., fresh fruit and vegetables, and well-cooked pulses, and avoids white flour and refined sugar, is assured of plenty of fibre to protect him against fibre-related diseases.

## SALT – AN UNNECESSARY HABIT

Salt (sodium chloride) and sugar are probably the most harmful single substances present in a child's diet, taking into account the amounts consumed. Excessive salt intake often begins when well-meaning mothers over-concentrate dried infant formula, or start solid food too soon. This may damage the highly sensitive infant kidneys. Breast milk contains the 'ideal' amount of salt and cannot become over-concentrated. After four months of age a baby's kidneys are mature enough to begin to handle small amounts of added salt.

It has been shown, however, that salt consumption is the main dietary factor which influences the development of high blood pressure in later life. High blood pressure is the largest single cause of death in this country, and many young children will become potential victims in adulthood because of the dangerous salt levels in their diets of snacks and convenience foods. Very salty food may also cause stomach cancer.

Since salt appetite is unrelated to salt requirements, and is perhaps a learned phenomenon, restriction of salt intake from infancy may be considered as a contribution to a reduction in the incidence of high blood pressure in later life. It is much easier to restrict salt intake in babies and young children than to reverse an acquired salt appetite at a later stage.

Salt may legally be added to baby foods. It is also added to a wide range of products including most children's breakfast cereals, bread, butter, cheese and almost all canned and processed foods. Some mothers also habitually add salt to the meals they prepare for their children, because they think they taste too bland.

## VITAMINS – DEFICIENCY AND TOXICITY

Vitamins are the organic constituents of common foods which are needed for proper growth and to give protection against disease. When food is processed, many essential nutrients are lost. They are either damaged by heating or are lost because they are present in those parts of the food which are removed during processing. It is possible that a young child eating a diet largely consisting of highly refined foods – white sugar, white flour, junk foods, etc. – and overcooked foods may suffer from lack of one or more vitamins.

Refined sugar and highly sweetened foods are particularly dangerous as they provide 'empty' calories.

Fortunately, as a result of the wide variety and sheer quantity of food that is consumed, overt deficiency diseases, such as scurvy and beriberi, are now rare in this country. Rickets, however, a childhood disease due to lack of vitamin D, in which the bones are softened and deformed, is still a problem among certain population groups. The DHSS recognizes the needs of babies and young children for vitamin D and recommends that babies should receive either Children's Vitamin Drops containing vitamins A, C and D (available from child health clinics), or another source of vitamin D, by the time they are one month old. This should be continued until the child is at least two and preferably until five years of age. A vitamin D supplement is particularly important for children eating a wholefood diet, as fibre increases requirements for this vitamin.

Many mothers, through ignorance, are not seeing that their children receive these vital supplements, and although few children will develop recognizable rickets (bow legs, knock knees) as a result, they may not achieve as good a bone structure as they might. Poor bone structure affects a child's appearance – especially his teeth – since a jaw which does not grow adequately will cause the mouth to be overcrowded and ugly. Outward appearance seems to affect the way people relate to each other, and it would seem that concern in this area is long overdue.

Vitamin toxicity (poisoning) may occur if too large an amount is taken. This is almost unknown when the vitamin is taken as part of a wholefood and normally only results from over-zealous consumption of commercial vitamin preparations. Vitamins A and D are particularly liable to cause toxicity when taken in excess.

## MINERAL DEFICIENCY

Minerals are essential nutrients which must be supplied in the diet. The most common childhood condition related to mineral deficiency in the West is undoubtedly iron-deficiency anaemia. Millions of children suffer from this complaint and it could be prevented if enough dietary iron were consumed. Children in the West who are faddy eaters may not consume enough iron-rich food, and that which they do get may not be absorbed owing to other factors in the diet. Tea, for example, inhibits iron absorption and so does a lack of vitamin C (from fresh fruits, etc.).

Goitre is another mineral deficiency disease seen among Western children, and is due to lack of iodine in the environment. This can be prevented by eating foods known to be rich in this mineral, such as seafood or fish-liver oils. There are many other conditions relating to deficiencies of certain minerals in the diet. They are rarely seen, however, in children eating a healthy diet.

## FOOD ADDITIVES – HOW HARMFUL ARE THEY?

Children are exposed to a variety of additives whenever they eat food which has been highly processed. Additives were originally used to preserve food – salt and sugar – but nowadays one of their main uses is to make food more attractive by improving such qualities as flavour, colour and texture. It is not always realized that children's food tends to contain more additives than adults' food and, since children weigh less than adults, the toxic load on them is much greater.

The effect that chemical food additives may have on health is a hotly debated subject. Some additives, such as cyclamate (a sweetener), have been shown to be harmful in large doses and are now banned in this country, but for many other additives the evidence against their use is not so clear-cut. One particular additive which can be lethal to babies under sixteen weeks is sodium nitrate or nitrite. This is present in many preserved and canned foods such as ham and sausages. It may lead to poisoning similar to carbon monoxide poisoning. Nitrites can also form carcinogenic (cancer-forming) substances – nitrosamines – in the body.

Another additive which is best avoided, although present in almost all savoury snacks, is monosodium glutamate (MSG). It contributes to the sodium content of the diet and causes unpleasant symptoms in some sensitive people.

Food additives are becoming increasingly implicated in many allergic conditions. Both eczema and asthma respond to additive-free diets in many cases, as do some cases of hyperactivity among children.

A long-term and more serious side effect of additives is their possible carcinogenicity. New additives are tested on animals to see if they cause cancer. Animal studies, however, cannot always be extrapolated to man and the interaction between many different additives present in one product has not been studied. It is reasonable to assume that most additives, being unnatural substances, are bound to have a deleterious effect on health. Indeed, additives formerly in common use have been banned in the UK after animal studies have shown them to be carcinogenic. Some colourings banned in Europe or the USA continue to be permitted in the UK.

## ENVIRONMENTAL HAZARDS

By carefully reading the labels on packaged foods, one can get a reasonable idea of what they contain. There are many unwanted non-nutritious substances, however, whose presence is not declared. These are the neurotoxic metals, such as lead, mercury and cadmium, and also the pesticides and radioactivity present in all foods to a greater or lesser degree. Other hazards include the microorganisms with which unwrapped food often becomes contaminated due to poor storage or lack of hygiene during handling.

All these hidden toxins can cause disease, either immediately or during adulthood, and an attempt should be made to remove or avoid them as far as possible. This involves carefully washing or peeling whole grains, fruits and vegetables to remove, as much as possible, external contamination from pesticides and airborne metals such as lead. Foods which children should avoid are principally from those animals and plants which are known to contain high levels of toxins. These include all shellfish, fish which have lived in areas of high radioactivity, certain Pacific fish such as tuna which contain high levels of mercury, and fruit and vegetables grown near busy roads.

# FOOD FACTS

The three basic nutrients – protein, carbohydrate and fat – stand quite apart from other requirements of the body, such as vitamins and minerals, since they are needed in much larger quantities; they are the fuel and building materials which are used in bulk. While daily requirements of vitamins and minerals are recorded in amounts that can be measured in milligrams or even micrograms (a thousandth of a milligram), protein, carbohydrate and fat intakes are expressed in grams, which is to say they are needed in amounts one thousand to one million times as great.

Protein is the basic building block of the body. If more protein is eaten than is needed, and if the intake of carbohydrate is low, the body will tend to burn the extra protein as fuel.

The carbohydrates – sugar and starch – provide the fuel on which the body runs and comprise the bulk of the diet. Although the body can burn fats or proteins, it does not do so as efficiently as it burns carbohydrates, so for smooth physiological functioning, substantial quantities of carbohydrate are constantly used. The body can convert excess carbohydrate into fat, which is essentially a storage form of fuel. This can later be burned when there is no ready source of carbohydrate. Animals also make and store fat, and when animal foods (meat, fish, etc.) are eaten, fat becomes a significant part of the diet.

Plants make some fats too, the majority of which tend to have a low melting point and are therefore normally encountered in liquid form – oil. Certain of these oils (essential fatty acids), which are much more plentiful in plants than in animals, cannot be manufactured and are essential to a healthy diet in small amounts. Otherwise fat in the adult diet is taken less out of necessity than out of preference. Babies and young children, however, have special needs for fat.

The normal diet contains more fat than protein and more carbo-hydrate than fat. Most wholefoods – grains, pulses, fruits and vegetables – with the exception of meat and fish flesh, which contains no carbohydrate, contain a balance of the three major nutrients as well as appropriate amounts of vitamins and minerals. Only with the coming of modern technology has man been able to separate out cheaply and easily the basic nutrients, yielding rela-tively pure fat or carbohydrate, for example, and creating the 'refined' foods, mineral and vitamin pills that are increasingly available today. This provides both the possibility of quickly sup-plying that which is deficient and the danger of taking excessive amounts of one of these nutrients. It also presents the hazard of disrupting the balance in food that nature offers, thereby destroying the equilibrium of a natural diet. This can cause a variety of health problems, as will be explained later.

## PROTEIN

A protein molecule is a long chain whose links are the smaller nitrogen-containing units called amino acids. Most of the twenty amino acid molecules can be converted into others, or manufac-tured by the body if there is a shortage of one type. There are nine, however, which a child's body cannot synthesize in this way and they must be taken in the diet already formed. These are called the 'essential amino acids'. The nitrogen from excess protein in the diet is eventually converted to urea – a relatively harmless substance which is filtered out of the bloodstream by the kidneys and excreted into the urine. The carbon, hydrogen and oxygen fraction is used to supply energy.

Protein is needed for growth, and during adulthood there is a decreasing requirement for it. Skin, hair, nails, cartilage, tendons, muscles and even the organic framework of bones are made up largely of proteins. Protein is needed to replace tissues that are continually breaking down, and to build up tissues, such as hair and nails, which are continually growing. The body depends on protein for many different purposes; some hormones such as insulin are proteins, and so are enzymes – the biological catalysts.

Haemoglobin, the critical oxygen-carrying molecule of the blood, is built from protein, and blood proteins help prevent excess alka-linity or acidity, maintaining the 'body neutrality' essential to normal cellular metabolism. They also help to regulate the body's water balance, the distribution of fluid on either side of the cell membrane. New protein synthesis is needed to form antibodies to fight bacterial and viral infections. Protein can also be converted into carbohydrate and used to provide energy, 1 g of dietary protein supplying 4 kcal (17 kJ) of energy. The body needs a daily supply of protein in order to maintain health as, unlike carbohydrate or fat, there are no significant reserves of it.

Animal foods – meat, fish, cheese, milk and eggs – are traditionally considered to be 'protein foods', but there are many important plant sources of protein. These include beans, peas and lentils, especially soya beans; whole grains, such as wheat, oats and rice; and nuts and seeds. Even green and most root vegetables contain significant amounts of protein. Fruit and butter contain a small amount, and sugar, oil and honey none. Heat alters the structure of protein, and when cooking times are prolonged or temperatures are extreme, it will become less available for utilization within the body.

PROTEIN COMPLEMENTARITY

Animal protein is generally of a higher quality and more useful to the body than plant protein, because all of the essential amino acids are present in approximately ideal proportions. Plant foods do not have such a well-balanced amino acid content and so are less usable. More poor-quality protein than good-quality protein must be eaten to fulfil the daily requirements for essential amino acids.

Nutritionists in the past believed that if no milk, meat or eggs were eaten, one would eventually die from lack of adequate protein. It is now known that the grains, pulses or vegetables in traditional diets are rarely eaten alone, but are taken in combination, so that the amino acids absent in one are supplied by those present in another. This is possible because the deficiencies of the essential amino acids are different for beans, for grains and for vegetables. Grains can therefore be combined with pulses – baked beans on toast, for example – to improve the quality of the protein. Their amino acids are said to be complementary, since what each lacks the other supplies. Such protein mixes do not result in a perfect protein that is fully utilizable by the body (only egg is near perfect), but combinations will increase the protein quality by as much as 50 per cent above the average of the items when eaten separately.

Even when plant foods are eaten alone and not in combination, there is little danger to adults of protein deficiency, as most foods contain some protein even though it may be of poor quality. Protein deficiency, however, may occur on diets heavily dependent on fruits (fruitarian diets), or on tubers such as sweet potatoes and cassava, which often happens in the areas of the Third World where chronic food shortages are present.

Uncomplemented plant diets cannot be recommended for babies or young children because not only do they need a diet richer in protein than that eaten by adults, but they cannot digest certain plant foods as easily. Special care is therefore required in meeting their needs if a largely plant-food diet only is available.

There are four principal food groups whose proteins when eaten in combination may complement each other and so increase the overall quality. These are grains (wheat, rye, barley, oats, rice, maize), seeds (sesame and sunflower), pulses (beans, peas and lentils) and milk products. Grains and milk products, grains and pulses, and seeds and pulses are the food combinations where complementary protein relationships have been confirmed. A complementary relationship has only been demonstrated in very few items in the following groups: grains and seeds, seeds and milk products, and pulses and milk products. Here are some examples of dishes popular with children where the proteins complement each other and so form good-quality protein:

*Grains and pulses*

Baked beans on wholemeal toast
Brown rice and bean casserole
Pea soup and bread
Bean soup and bread

*Grains and milk products*

Rice pudding
Wholewheat spaghetti with cheese
  sauce
Cereal and milk
Macaroni cheese
Cheese sandwiches

*Seeds and pulses*

Sunflower seeds and peanuts
  (pulses)
Hummus and tahina (chick peas
  and sesame)

*Grains and seeds*

Toast or bread with sesame or
  sunflower spread
Rice or bread with sesame seeds

*Seeds and milk products*

Sesame and milk

*Pulses and milk products*

Bean and milk soup

Contrary to popular belief, a diet containing adequate protein need not be expensive. It is not necessary for the child to have costly foods such as meat, fish, nuts and cheese. Eggs, milk, pulses and cereals, at the cheaper end of the scale, will provide the daily protein requirement at very little cost.

HOW MUCH PROTEIN DO CHILDREN NEED?

A toddler is adequately served by 30 g of protein per day. The amount of protein present in 100 g (3½ oz) portions of some basic foods rich in protein is as follows:

> 4 tablespoons cooked beef stewing steak     31 g
> 3 heaped tablespoons grilled cod     21 g
> 2 eggs (size 4)     12 g
> 100 g (3½ oz) Cheddar cheese     26 g
> 5 tablespoons dry lentils     24 g
> 5 tablespoons peanuts     24 g
> 100 ml (⅙ pt) milk     3 g
> 6 heaped tablespoons wholemeal flour     13 g

The recommended protein allowances are, however, calculated for healthy people. Ill health may lead to increased requirements. Stress, such as pain, can push up the need for protein by as much as one third. Since most children eat far more protein than they can use, they can easily obtain the 'extra' protein needed when under stress from that already in their diets. Other stress situations include an inadequate energy (calorie) intake. Some dietary protein is then used for energy and so is not available for growth and tissue repair. Infections, especially acute ones, cause a loss of body nitrogen and these losses need to be replaced with additional protein during recovery.

By observing the child, it is easy to judge if his protein needs are being met. Many types of minor nutritional deficiencies show up as deterioration in the hair, skin and nails and in the slow healing of wounds. Except during early infancy, a moderate excess of protein has not been shown to be harmful.

## CARBOHYDRATE

Though many other nutrients have since been discovered, in terms of sheer quantity carbohydrate remains the most important. The average person eats 100 g of carbohydrate for every 10 g of protein. Starches and sugars are carbohydrates and so is cellulose – the most abundant carbohydrate in nature. Cellulose and other undigested polysaccharides contribute to the dietary fibre.

During digestion, starches and dextrins – formed when starch is subjected to dry heat – are split to their component units of glucose; sucrose (table sugar) to its component units of glucose and fructose; lactose (milk sugar) to its component units of glucose and galactose. These simple sugars are absorbed into the bloodstream and either stored for later use in the form of fat or glycogen (long sugar chains), or used immediately for energy. It is on this energy that all metabolism depends. Glucose and sugar are not superior sources of energy – all carbohydrates contain 3.75 kcal (16 kJ) per gram – although they may be absorbed into the bloodstream at a faster rate than proteins or fats.

SUGAR (simple carbohydrate)

Most of the sugar in the diet of primitive man was found in fruit. The sweetness of the fruit enticed him to eat it; he then carried the seed with him and deposited it elsewhere, so propagating the growth and spread of the plant species. The sugar in modern diets, however, is most likely to be the white substance made by refining sugar cane or sugar beet. Sucrose, glucose, fructose, maltose and lactose are all sugars, although the word sugar is commonly taken to mean table sugar (sucrose).

Pure white sugar contains no protein, no vitamins, no minerals and no fat or fibre. It is a stripped carbohydrate and consists essentially of 'empty' calories; it can be cut out of the diet completely without any penalty. Nutritionally speaking, when sugar is eaten a 'debt' is incurred. Though the need for carbohydrate has been met, the body is owed a corresponding quantity of vitamins, minerals, fat, protein and fibre. Furthermore, the metabolism of the sugar itself requires vitamins, minerals and even some protein and fat. This is why in diets containing a lot of sugar, obesity and malnutrition may occur together. Under a mountain of fat, many obese people are starving to death because they are not getting enough essential nutrients. The over-consumption of sugar is directly responsible for many modern diseases, particularly heart disease and diabetes. Even brown sugar is a highly purified product and is just as harmful as white.

Although most of the sugar in the diet is usually the refined variety, many wholefoods – particularly fruits – contain significant amounts of natural sugars. These natural sugars are not as harmful to health as the purified, refined sugars, as they are only eaten in very small quantities at a time – it is difficult to eat too many apples. Furthermore, they come packaged with a balanced complement of the other nutrients required by the body.

Honey is a very complex substance consisting of about 23 per cent water and about 76 per cent sugars – mostly fructose and glucose – with only traces of other nutrients. The quality of honey depends on its origin and how it is made. When used as a sweetener in the diet, honey has a slight advantage over sugar in that it contains fewer calories and, as it is sweeter than sugar, less is needed. Honey is, however, a concentrated sugar and, other than in small amounts, is best avoided.

While there are disadvantages to concentrated sugars of all kinds, there is clearly a need for carbohydrate in the diet. A certain amount of fuel must be burned each day and if sufficient carbohydrate is not eaten, the body must turn to the use of fat or proteins. Neither of these burns well, especially in the absence of carbohydrates, and the residues they produce can cause problems. Therefore a form of carbohydrate other than simple sugars is required.

STARCH (complex carbohydrate)

Starch – a polysaccharide – is a complex carbohydrate. Its large branched chains are formed by many sugar molecules linked together. In the last hundred years the total carbohydrate consumption has decreased, probably because increased mechanization has resulted in less physical work for the average person. The drop in carbohydrate consumption is due to the dramatic fall in consumption of complex carbohydrates found in grains and beans, since the use of simple carbohydrates, like table sugar, has more than doubled.

Starch is essentially the storage form of carbohydrate which plants use in much the same way as animals use fat. It is starch that nourishes the plant during the early stages of its development before it establishes a root and leaf system for manufacturing its own nourishment. It is therefore 'packaged' along with the other critical nutrients – vitamins, minerals and proteins – that will be needed during its growth. Starch is dismantled by enzymes during digestion and the liberated glucose is absorbed into the bloodstream.

Though some carbohydrate is present in the leaves and stems of plants, man and many animals depend for the bulk of their fuel on certain seeds. Throughout the world, seeds or 'grains' are the most valued source of starch. Cereals contain about 70 per cent starch, bread 50 per cent, chestnuts 30 per cent, potatoes 20 per cent, pulses 10–15 per cent, other nuts and root vegetables up to 5 per cent. Leaves and fruits contain traces.

When starch is refined, pure (edible) starch is obtained. This is extensively used by the food industry as a thickener and stabilizer. Arrowroot, sago, tapioca and cornflour are virtually pure starch, which is essentially a stripped carbohydrate. It provides 'empty' calories, failing, like sugar, to bring with it the necessary complement of vitamins, minerals and proteins that are needed to carry on the metabolism that it could energize, and 'spoiling' the appetite for nutritious foods. Most convenience foods, including baby foods, contain 'modified' starch and are, for this reason, best avoided.

HOW MUCH CARBOHYDRATE DO CHILDREN NEED?

There is no recommended intake for carbohydrate in the diet because fats and proteins also supply energy to the body. The bulk of the diet does, however, normally consist of carbohydrate-rich foods, owing to their wide availability and cheapness. If energy in the form of carbohydrate and fat is low, protein is wasted, as it will be burned for energy rather than used for rebuilding. Almost all the carbohydrate in a child's diet should be unrefined – wholegrain cereals, pulses, vegetables and fruit – rather than refined carbohydrates present in sweets, soft drinks, jams, ice cream, instant desserts and so on, which provide energy but little else, and rob the body of the nutrients which are needed to metabolize them.

FATS

Although generally used to describe concentrated fatty foods like fat on meat, and separated fat like butter, the term 'fat' applies equally to the non-visible fat to be found in nearly all foods. Even lean roast beef and eggs, for instance, contain about 12 per cent of their weight as fat, peanuts about half.

Fats are solid at low temperatures – lard, for example – and become liquid when heated. Oils are simply fats which are liquid at room temperature, usually as a result of their higher content of unsaturated fatty acids. Most animals tend to store their energy as saturated fats, while plants and fish tend to store their energy as unsaturated 'oils'. Highly unsaturated fats are called polyunsaturated fatty acids (PUFA).

Nearly all fat in the diet is composed of 'triglycerides' or simple fats. These are formed by the attachment of three fatty acids to a neutral compound called glycerol. Polyunsaturated fatty acids with a chemical structure that cannot be imitated by the body, are essential to our health. Linoleic acid – mainly found in vegetable oils and chicken fat – is the most important of this group and must be taken in the diet. All other fatty acids can be synthesized by the body and are not essential nutrients.

Fat makes an important contribution to the texture and palatability of foods, and because it is digested comparatively slowly, foods rich in fat have a high satiety value. Animal fats may contain vitamins A and D and varying amounts of cholesterol, while vegetable fats may contain carotenes (which can be converted into vitamin A in the body) and vitamin E, but no cholesterol. All saturated fats, whether they come from animal or vegetable sources, raise blood cholesterol.

Fat is the highest energy-yielding nutrient, supplying 9 kcal (37 kJ) per gram. Foods which are nearly all fat – like vegetable oils – provide more energy, weight for weight, than any other food.

Animals, including man, store excess energy almost entirely in deposits of fat, the amount of which is very variable. As in plants, this fat can be made from carbohydrates, but the dietary carbohydrate can be starch, sugar, or even – in cows and sheep – fibre. Animals also lay down fat from the fat they eat.

There are many sources of fat in the diet. Butter, lard, Cheddar cheese, beef and most other meats are high in fat. So are fish such as herring, mackerel, pilchards, salmon, sardine, tuna and eels. White fish such as cod, haddock and plaice contain little fat except in the liver. In plants, fats are formed from carbohydrate. Thus, when seeds such as sunflower and cottonseed ripen, their starch content decreases as their fat content rises. Oil seeds such as these, and groundnuts (peanuts), coconuts, rape, palm and soya beans contain about 20–40 per cent oil; they are among the chief sources of fat for the manufacture of margarines. The fat content of flour and other cereal products, apart from oatmeal, is generally low, as is the fat content of most vegetables and fruit. Sugar is fat-free.

Some fat-like substances in the body are different from the simple carbon chains that make up most oils and animal fats. The best-known of these is cholesterol. Not a triglyceride, it is a waxy fat-like compound which serves a multitude of purposes in the body. Cholesterol is essential to life. It is a building block of the outer membrane of cells, and is a principal ingredient in the digestive juice bile, in the fatty sheath that insulates nerves and in sex hormones. Although most of the cholesterol found in the body is produced in the liver, 20–30 per cent generally comes from the diet. Foods very high in cholesterol include egg yolk, fish roe, offal, butter and double cream. Meat (both lean and fat), fish and most cheeses contain moderate amounts. Vegetables, vegetable oils, fruit and cereals contain none.

Lecithins are the main phospholipids (emulsifiers) in the blood-stream and are concerned with the transport of fat – cholesterol, for example – about the body. They can be made in the body and are not essential nutrients. They are found in most foods; egg yolks are the richest source.

Mineral oils such as liquid paraffin are chemically different from food fats and oils, despite their similarity in appearance. They cannot be utilized by the body, but function as laxatives and reduce the absorption of vitamins A, D, E and K. They are added to some foods – dried fruit, citrus fruit, sweets and chewing gum – and small amounts may be absorbed and deposited in the liver. Impurities are suspected carcinogens.

HOW MUCH FAT DO CHILDREN NEED?

In adulthood, there appears to be no absolute dietary requirement for fat, except for a small amount (1–2 per cent of energy requirements) of essential fatty acids. Their lack leads to growth retardation, skin changes with hair loss, increase in metabolic rate and early death. Rich sources of these fatty acids include sunflower-seed oil, soya-bean oil, corn (maize) oil, groundnut (peanut) oil and peanut butter. Animal foods contain little, except for chicken fat, which contains a moderate amount. Some scientists now believe that the optimum intake of essential fatty acids should be much higher than the amount that prevents deficiency disease, in order to protect against heart and blood-vessel disease.

A substantial amount of fat is, however, required in childhood, particularly in infancy, when the need for calories is high. If fat were not added to formula feeds, for example, then the volume of feed would need to be increased, as energy requirements per unit weight are at their highest. Fat increases the palatability of the diet and is a vehicle for fat-soluble vitamins. After the age of two, fat intakes should be, on average, one third of the total energy intake. If, however, a large part of the diet consists of fatty foods such as crisps, chips, hamburgers and sausages, the proportion of fat will be much higher than this.

Excessive fat consumption constitutes a major health risk, even to young children, as it may lead to early furring-up of the arteries and eventual heart disease. Obesity with its many associated problems is also related to high fat intake.

## VITAMINS

Although it had been known for some time that certain foods were protective against diseases like scurvy and beriberi, it was believed that the only components of a diet necessary for health, growth and reproduction were pure proteins, carbohydrates, fats and a number of inorganic elements. This view had to be changed when it was found that minute amounts of additional materials were also essential. These materials could be extracted from a variety of foods, and appeared to be of two types: fat-soluble and water-soluble. They were later each discovered to contain several active components or vitamins.

Fat-soluble vitamins, mainly associated with fatty foods, are now known to include vitamins A, D, E and K. The water-soluble vitamins include both the B complex and vitamin C. Fat-soluble vitamins are more stable to cooking and processing than the B vitamins and vitamin C, which leach out of foods into cooking water, and are often readily destroyed by heat. Humans are known to require thirteen different vitamins, which have different functions and occur in a wide range of foods.

### Vitamin A (retinol)

Vitamin A was one of the first vitamins to be discovered. It is a fat-soluble vitamin and essential for many body functions, particularly the health of the skin, and also for the 'inner skin' – the membranes that line the breathing system, lungs, ears and bladder.

Vitamin A is not widely distributed in food. Fish-liver oils are by far the most concentrated natural source, but animal liver, kidney, dairy produce and eggs also contain substantial amounts. Variable amounts of carotene – a substance from which the body can make retinol – are found in milk and also in carrots, and dark green or yellow vegetables and fruit, roughly in proportion to the depth of their colour. Dark plants such as spinach, therefore contain more than lighter ones such as cabbage, and the dark outer leaves of cabbage may contain fifty times as much as the inner white ones. All margarine is required by law to contain about the same amount of vitamin A as does butter. Cereals, nuts, meat, white fish, white vegetables and fruit, oils (except red palm oil) and white fats contain virtually no vitamin A.

The main sources of vitamin A in the diet are butter, margarine, liver, milk, green vegetables and carrots. Vitamin A in food can be destroyed by prolonged exposure to light, frying and drying. Milk left on the doorstep, for instance, loses some vitamin A.

HOW MUCH VITAMIN A DO CHILDREN NEED?

Babies receive ample vitamin A from breast milk or fortified infant formula. After weaning, however, care should be taken to ensure that adequate vitamin A is obtained. The recommended daily intake of vitamin A is 450 µg (retinol equivalents) for babies less than 1 year of age and 300 µg for children aged 1–5 years.* The amount of vitamin A present in 100 g (3½ oz) portions of some basic foods rich in this vitamin is as follows:

    100 ml (⅙ pt) milk    40 µg
    100 g (3½ oz) Cheddar cheese    412 µg
    1 large slice fried lamb's liver    20,610 µg
    4 tablespoons winter cabbage (boiled for 15 minutes)    50 µg
    1 medium raw carrot    2,000 µg
    4 tablespoons dried apricots    600 µg

Children's Vitamin Drops or cod-liver oil contain vitamin A as well as vitamin D and guarantee a child's daily requirements. The stated dose should not be exceeded.

Without enough vitamin A, the skin becomes rough and dry, with

---

* 1,000 µg (micrograms) = 1 mg (milligram).

dead cells blocking the glands through which the natural oils travel to lubricate the smooth skin surface. The hair too will lack sheen and the scalp will be dry and clogged with dead cells. The same process affects the eyes. In the Third World, deficiency of vitamin A is a widespread cause of blindness. In the West, this degree of deficiency is very rare – but it is quite possible to lack enough vitamin A to make it difficult to see well in dim light.

Excessive doses, for example from taking large amounts of vitamin A preparations for long periods, accumulate in the liver and can be toxic. This is less likely to happen, however, when oil-based preparations, e.g. cod-liver oil, are given.

## B vitamins

The eight B vitamins known to be essential nutrients for humans are generally classified as the B complex. In the young of most species a lack of any vitamins of the B complex results in poor growth and a failure to thrive. Although the chemical structures of each of the B vitamins is quite different, they have several features in common. They act as 'co-factors' in different enzyme systems in the body, and tend to occur in the same foods. Being water-soluble, they are not stored for long in the body. These characteristics mean that diets containing too little of the B vitamins can lead to multiple deficiency diseases within a few months.

Originally, the germ of cereals was thought to contain only one vitamin – the anti-beriberi vitamin or vitamin B. Later on, others were discovered and numbered vitamin $B_1$ to vitamin $B_{12}$. Some, however, were later found not to be vitamins or had already been discovered. As a result, only four B complex vitamins are still numbered, $B_1$ (thiamin), $B_2$ (riboflavin), $B_6$ (pyridoxine), and vitamin $B_{12}$.

### THIAMIN (vitamin $B_1$)

Thiamin is necessary for the steady and continuous release of energy from carbohydrate. Thiamin requirements are thus related to the amount of carbohydrate in the diet and, more or less, to the amount of energy used.

Thiamin is widely distributed in both animal and vegetable foods. Rich sources are yeast, milk, offal, pork, eggs, vegetables and fruit, wholegrain cereals and fortified breakfast cereals. Fats and sugars contain no thiamin. White bread is fortified with this vitamin. The main sources of thiamin in the diet are bread and flour, meat, potatoes and milk. Cooking in an excess of water may result in considerable losses of thiamin if the water is discarded. Baking powder also destroys thiamin.

The deficiency disease, beriberi, results from a diet which is not only poor in thiamin but also rich in carbohydrate, such as one based almost entirely on polished rice from which the thiamin-rich seed coat has been removed. Beriberi is primarily a disease affecting the brain and nerves, but it is rare in Britain, except amongst alcoholics. Thiamin is not stored in the body and excess thiamin is lost rapidly in the urine.

## RIBOFLAVIN (vitamin $B_2$)

Riboflavin is a bright yellow substance which is essential for the utilization of energy from food.

It is widely distributed in foods, especially animal foods. About one third of the average intake in Britain is derived from milk. Natex low-salt yeast extract, Cheddar cheese, eggs, beef, chicken, liver and potatoes also contain significant amounts of riboflavin. Riboflavin is destroyed by ultraviolet light, and milk should not be allowed to stay too long on the doorstep. It may also be lost in cooking water. Riboflavin deficiency in man is rare; symptoms include sores in the corners of the mouth. Large doses of synthetic riboflavin do not appear to have adverse effects.

## NICOTINIC ACID

Nicotinic acid and nicotinamide are two forms of another B vitamin (known as niacin in the United States) which is involved in the utilization of energy from food. The main sources of nicotinic acid in the diet are meat and meat products, bread and flour, fortified breakfast cereals, vegetables and milk. Although it leaches out of food into cooking water, it is one of the most stable B vitamins and commercial processing and storage cause little loss. Deficiency results in a condition known as pellagra, in which the skin becomes dark and scaly, especially where it is exposed to light. Large amounts of synthetic nicotinic acid cause transient flushing, burning and tingling.

## VITAMIN $B_6$ (pyridoxine)

Vitamin $B_6$, or pyridoxine, is involved in the metabolism of amino acids; the requirements are thus related to the protein content of the diet. The vitamin is also necessary for the formation of haemoglobin.

Vitamin $B_6$ occurs in many foods, especially in meat and fish, eggs, wholegrain cereals and some vegetables. It is vulnerable to heat.

Deficiency is rare because of the wide distribution of the vitamin in food. The toxicity of synthetic pyridoxine is low.

### VITAMIN $B_{12}$

Vitamin $B_{12}$ is a mixture of several related compounds, all containing the trace element cobalt. With folic acid, it is needed by rapidly dividing cells such as those in the bone marrow which form blood.

Liver is the richest source, but useful amounts occur in eggs, cheese, milk, meat and fish, and it is manufactured by many bacteria and yeasts. Any food which is strictly of plant origin, not fermented, and free of all bacteria and insects, will be found to contain no vitamin $B_{12}$. Vitamin $B_{12}$ is fairly stable to heat but leaches out of food cooked in water.

Because vitamin $B_{12}$ does not occur in vegetable foods, deficiency may occur in vegans who consume no meat, milk or eggs, and do not take any special supplement, but it more usually arises in those few individuals whose gastric juice contains none of the 'intrinsic factor' necessary for its absorption. Deficiency results in anaemia. Excess vitamin $B_{12}$ is stored in the liver, but large doses are not toxic as little of the vitamin is absorbed into the bloodstream.

### FOLIC ACID

Folic acid has several functions, including its action with vitamin $B_{12}$ in rapidly dividing cells. It occurs in many foods – offal and raw green leafy vegetables are particularly good sources. Pulses, bread, oranges and bananas also provide folic acid, but other fruits, meat and dairy products contain little. Goats' milk is a very poor source of folate and 'goats' milk anaemia' is a recognized result of folate deficiency.

Food preparation can cause serious losses of folic acid – in prolonged heating, in canning, when cooking water is discarded, and from reheating. Vitamin C protects against the destruction of folic acid, however. Folic acid is not always well absorbed, and care should be taken to include good sources of this vitamin in the diet.

Deficiency leads to a characteristic form of anaemia. Folic-acid deficiency can arise not only from a poor diet, but also because of increased needs for the synthesis of red blood cells, in pregnant women and premature infants, for instance, or when there is decreased absorption of folic acid in gastro-intestinal disease, or when some anti-epileptic drugs are given. Excess folic acid is normally harmless – it is filtered out of the bloodstream by the kidneys.

PANTOTHENIC ACID

Pantothenic acid is necessary for the release of energy from fat and carbohydrate. Animal products, wholegrain cereals and pulses are especially rich sources. In most cooking and baking procedures there is little loss of the vitamin. Dietary deficiencies of this vitamin are unlikely in man because it is so widespread in food.

BIOTIN

Biotin is essential for the metabolism of fat. Rich sources of biotin include offal and egg yolk. Smaller amounts are obtained from milk and dairy products, cereals, fish, fruit and vegetables. Human milk has a naturally low content of biotin, and the seborrhoeic dermatitis (cradle cap) sometimes observed in infants with persistent diarrhoea is believed to result from a low intake of biotin coupled with excessive losses.

Very small amounts of biotin are required by the body and sufficient may well be made by the micro-organisms normally inhabiting the large intestine. It is therefore probable that no additional biotin need be provided by foods unless large quantities of raw egg are consumed, since raw, but not cooked, egg white contains a substance (avidin) which combines with biotin making it unavailable to the body.

HOW MUCH VITAMIN B DO CHILDREN NEED?

Children eating a nutritious mixed diet which includes fresh fruit and vegetables will obtain adequate amounts of all the B vitamins, if care is taken not to overcook food or discard cooking water.

Those foods which are rich in one member of the B complex are very likely to be rich in several of the others. The richest source of these vitamins is the germ and the bran of seeds such as cereals, nuts, beans, peas and so on. Leafy green vegetables and cows' milk are also good sources; so are some meats, such as pork, while others, such as beef, contain very little. Liver of almost any kind tends to contain high quantities of the B vitamins and is one of the richest sources. Yeast extract is also rich in B vitamins but most brands (e.g. Marmite) contain too much salt and are unsuitable for children. 'Low-salt' extracts are now available.

### Vitamin C (ascorbic acid)

Vitamin C is a water-soluble vitamin. Small amounts of vitamin C in the diet are essential for the maintenance of healthy connective tissue. Man is one of the few animals (along with monkeys and the guinea-pig) unable to form his own vitamin C, and he must therefore obtain it from food.

Vitamin C is not widely distributed in foods. Small amounts occur in milk – especially breast milk – and liver, but virtually all the vitamin C in most diets is derived from fruit and vegetables. Rich sources of vitamin C include blackcurrants, strawberries, mustard and cress, parsley, spinach, turnip tops, Brussels sprouts, cabbage and cauliflower. Good sources include oranges, lemons, grapefruit, tangerines, bean sprouts, new potatoes, tomatoes, blackberries, parsnips, peas and turnips. Poor sources include apples, apricots, bananas, cherries, grapes, pears, plums, carrots, celery, mushrooms, onions and old potatoes.

The highest single contributor to vitamin C intake in Britain is the potato, for the large amounts eaten more than compensate for the comparatively low vitamin C content. The only vegetable foods containing no vitamin C are cereal grains (unless they are allowed to sprout) and dried peas and beans. Eggs, fats, most dairy foods, fish, nuts and meat contain none. Exceptions are liver, kidneys, fresh fish roe and unripe walnuts.

The vitamin C content of fresh foods is greatly affected by the type and variety of plant grown and also the soil, climate and maturity when harvested. Fruits and vegetables that have just been harvested contain more vitamin C than those that have been stored, because the soft tissues of harvested plants are alive and continue to use up the vitamin C accumulated during the growth of the plant. Losses are increased if vegetables are allowed to wilt or if they are damaged by frost or bruising.

Vitamin C is the nutrient most vulnerable to cooking and processing. It leaches out of food cooked in water and is rapidly destroyed by the oxygen in the air. This process is accelerated by heat, alkalis (e.g. baking soda) and iron and copper. It is also destroyed by an enzyme released from vegetable cells during peeling and chopping. For this reason, tomatoes, citrus fruits and other fruits which can be eaten without preparation are the most reliable sources of vitamin C.

To avoid undue losses of vitamin C, vegetables and fruit should not be crushed or finely chopped before cooking. Furthermore, they should not be put into cold water which is then brought to the boil, but into boiling water from which the oxygen has been driven off. When the food is cooked, it should not be kept hot longer than is absolutely necessary before serving, because this can destroy almost all the vitamin C.

Frozen, canned and dehydrated foods lose 10–30 per cent of the vitamins when they are blanched. Further losses of vitamin C from dehydrated foods are minimal as long as modern processes are used. If they are dried by prolonged exposure to the heat or the sun (e.g. raisins) they will contain no vitamin C.

HOW MUCH VITAMIN C DO CHILDREN NEED?

Breast milk and fortified infant formulas provide sufficient vitamin C. After weaning, children under five need 20 mg of vitamin C daily from the diet. The amount of vitamin C present in 100 g (3½ oz) portions of some basic foods rich in this vitamin is as follows:

     ½ large orange    50 mg
     4 heaped tablespoons mashed old potatoes    8 mg
     10–12 small Brussels sprouts boiled for 15 minutes    40 mg
     1 medium (5 cm) fresh tomato    20 mg

Fortified children's fruit syrups (blackcurrant, orange or rosehip, etc.) are good sources of vitamin C, but should nevertheless be avoided owing to the high concentration of sugar (glucose, sucrose, etc.) they contain. Children's Vitamin Drops provide vitamin C and will guarantee a child's daily requirements.

The need for vitamin C is increased by wounds repaired by scars – a form of connective tissue – and by infections such as colds. Requirements may also be increased by stress. Increased quantities of vitamin C are therefore to be recommended when recovering from surgery, for example.

Deficiency soon results in bleeding, especially from small blood vessels into the gums, and wounds heal more slowly. Scurvy follows, and if the deficiency is prolonged, death results. Although infant scurvy is now a rarity the world over, mild deficiencies may occur in infants who are given unsupplemented cows' milk preparations.

Large doses of vitamin C are rarely toxic, as excess is lost in the urine. Claims that extremely large amounts of vitamin C (10–100 times the recommended intake) prevent or cure colds and other minor ailments have little scientific basis, but may prove to have some justification.

### Vitamin D (cholecalciferol, ergocalciferol)

Vitamin D – a fat-soluble vitamin – is necessary for maintaining the level of calcium (and phosphorus) in the blood. It achieves this primarily by enhancing the absorption of dietary calcium from the intestine, and by helping to regulate the interchange of calcium between blood and bone.

Vitamin D is obtained both from the action of sunlight on a substance in the skin, and from the diet. Sunlight is by far the most important source for most adults, who will need little or no extra from food. Children, however, have especially high requirements for bone growth, and need to obtain sufficient dietary vitamin D as well as having exposure to the sun.

Few foods contain vitamin D. Fish-liver oils are the richest source. Notable sources include fatty fish (herrings, sardines) and eggs. Dairy foods (butter, milk, cheese) and liver contain very small quantities. Other foods – fruit, vegetables, cereals, other fish, fats, oils and meat – contain none. Margarine, some weaning foods and breakfast cereals are fortified with vitamin D.

Vitamin D is stable to heat and does not leach out of foods cooked in water. The only losses thought to occur in cooking and processing are through the removal of fat when milk is skimmed and fatty fish is grilled.

HOW MUCH VITAMIN D DO CHILDREN NEED?

When available, vitamin D is transferred from the mother during pregnancy. This store tides the infant over the few months after birth. Since not all babies, however, will be born with sufficient vitamin D stores, a dietary supplement should be provided as a precautionary measure; 7.5 µg of vitamin D is recommended for babies older than one month, and 10 µg for those older than one year. Breast-feeding does not protect against vitamin D deficiency and breast-fed babies should be given Children's Vitamin Drops (available from child health clinics) starting when they are one month old. Most infant formulas are fortified with adequate vitamin D, and a vitamin D supplement must not be given to bottle-fed babies.

After weaning, some vitamin D may be obtained from the diet, but few foods contain important amounts of this vitamin. The amount of vitamin D in 100 g (3½ oz) portions of some basic foods rich in this vitamin is as follows:

> 2 eggs (size 4)      1.75 µg
> 1 medium grilled herring      25.0 µg
> 4 sardines (canned)      7.5 µg
> 100 g (3½ oz) margarine      8.0 µg

Some weaning foods, breakfast cereals and milk products are fortified with vitamin D. One daily dose (but never more) of Children's Vitamin Drops, cod-liver oil (from six months) or a proprietary preparation of vitamin D will guarantee a child's daily requirements, and it should be continued until the child reaches the age of five. The instructions should be read carefully and the dosage should not be exceeded. Vitamin D supplements are particularly important for children who eat vegetarian diets, or diets rich in wholegrains and high-fibre (bran) cereals, since these diets lead to some wastage of this vitamin.

Babies and children who obtain too little vitamin D develop rickets – a disease in which the bones are softened and deformed as a result of failure to absorb calcium from the small intestine. There may be few physical signs at first, and the first symptoms in the young infant may be delayed development and muscle weakness rather than bone deformation. Wrist and ankle joints may be enlarged and are occasionally painful.

The effect of prolonged vitamin deficiency is a reduction in the rate of growth of the long bones. The bones are soft and cannot support the weight of the body. This leads to skeletal deformities which most frequently affect the long bones of the legs with the result that knock knees or bow legs may be formed. The rachitic child is a weakling with an increased risk of infections, especially respiratory ones.

Severe deformities such as these are uncommon nowadays in this country except among Asian and a small proportion of West Indian children. This is due to lack of utilization of welfare foods, to which additional risk factors, of dark skin, prolonged breast-feeding and vegetarian diets in later infancy may be added. In recent years the hazard of macrobiotic cult diets has been associated with multiple nutritional deficiencies, including rickets, in a very small number of white infants.

Milder forms of the disease are, however, more frequent than many people suppose. Symptoms include bone pain and muscle weakness, especially of the lower limbs. The effect of this weakness is to make it difficult for a child to rise from a sitting position without support from the arms. Because bone changes readily become permanent, it is important to prevent their development by giving children vitamin D supplements.

Even milder deficiencies of vitamin D during the years of rapid growth may result in deformities such as bulging or slanting foreheads, narrow little faces with overcrowded teeth, receding jaws, close-set eyes, hollow underdeveloped chests and inward curving backbones. One sees these unattractive features in a high proportion of children and as the child gets older these deformities become worse. Parents often believe these characteristics to be hereditary. While this is partly true, an optimal supply of vitamin D both from the diet and the sun can greatly influence a child's appearance.

Too high an intake of vitamin D causes more calcium to be absorbed from the diet than can be excreted; the excess is then deposited in the blood vessels, which can be fatal. It is therefore necessary for the vitamin D intake to be carefully controlled, especially in young children.

### Vitamin E (tocopherols)

The basic function of vitamin E remains the subject of much speculation – at one time it was assumed to act principally as an antioxidant, preventing damaging alteration to fat molecules in cells by oxygen – but this explanation has been criticized. Vitamin E is held in the membranes of cells, and is likely to be important in maintaining their structure.

There are at least eight substances in food which have vitamin E activity, the most active being alpha($\alpha$)-tocopherol. Although soluble in fat and found in fatty foods – vegetable oils are the richest source – vitamin E is also supplied by foods containing little fat (e.g. cereals, fish, fruit and vegetables). Rich sources are wheatgerm, most vegetable oils, olive oil and peanuts. Good sources include eggs, butter, cheese, wholemeal flour and bread, oats, carrots, cabbage, peas, plums and apples. Poor sources are white flour and bread, white and brown rice, refined breakfast cereals, most meat and fish, milk, oranges and bananas.

There are probably minimal losses of vitamin E in cooking – it is fairly stable to heat and does not leach out of foods cooked in water – but there may be severe losses in processing and storage. Wholemeal bread, for instance, is a good source of vitamin E, but much is removed with the germ during milling. Bleaching agents used in white flour destroy any remaining vitamin. Refined breakfast cereals contain little or no vitamin E. In fats, vitamin E acts as an antioxidant, preventing rancidity and preserving vitamin A, but eventually it is oxidized and becomes inactive. Rancid fats and oils contain none, neither do repeatedly used frying oils. Canned vegetables are reported to lose up to 90 per cent; there may be severe losses during prolonged deep-freeze storage.

HOW MUCH VITAMIN E DO CHILDREN NEED?

Requirements for vitamin E are provided by an adequate infant formula or breast milk. After weaning, deficiency is extremely rare as so many foods contain vitamin E. As long as a child is eating some vegetable oils, eggs, butter, cheese and wholemeal bread, he is unlikely to be lacking in this vitamin. It must be remembered, however, that polyunsaturated fat increases the need for this vitamin and individual needs may vary considerably.

Like other fat-soluble vitamins it is stored in the body, so deficiency is only likely in premature infants who have very low fat stores. This may happen if they are fed on a formula low in vitamin E and rich in the readily oxidized polyunsaturated fatty acids (vegetable oils). These appear to increase the need for this vitamin, and anaemia may develop as a result of increased destruction of red blood cells. Excessive intakes do not appear to be toxic.

## Vitamin K

Vitamin K is necessary for the normal clotting of blood. It is contained in vegetable foods and intestinal bacteria can synthesize it. Cabbage, sprouts, cauliflower and spinach are rich sources. Beans, peas, potatoes, carrots and beef liver are good sources. Losses of vitamin K in cooking and processing are thought to be minor.

Newborn babies are susceptible to vitamin K deficiency; in the first few days after birth they have no bacteria inhabiting the digestive system, and milk is a poor source. If bleeding does occur, a preparation of vitamin K is administered. Dietary deficiency is unlikely after the newborn period.

## MINERALS

Minerals are essential nutrients which must be supplied in the diet. They have three main functions. They may be incorporated into body structures such as bones and teeth, they may act as soluble salts which help to control the composition of body fluids and cells, or they may function as essential adjuncts to enzymes (co-factors). At least fifteen minerals are required by the body. Eight – calcium, phosphorus, sulphur, potassium, sodium, chlorine, magnesium and iron – are found in food and the body in relatively large quantities, by comparison with the minute amounts of the other minerals – the trace elements. These include fluorine, zinc, copper, iodine, manganese, chromium and cobalt.

Knowledge of the exact roles and dietary requirements for several of the trace elements is incomplete, for three reasons: they have only recently been found to be essential; dietary deficiency of many are unknown; and the utilization of one may be affected by the amounts of other elements present. Excess quantities of trace elements are toxic and there is often only a small difference between the quantity needed for health and the quantity which causes harm. The risk of obtaining too little or too much in food is minimized by eating a wide variety of foods in moderation. Food processing, changes in agricultural practices (such as excessive use of fertilizers, new breeds of plants) and changes in dietary habits (such as eating more fat in place of cereals) may alter the balance of trace elements in the diet.

These alterations may affect the development of some Western diseases, for instance heart disease. Cadmium, calcium, chromium, copper, selenium, vanadium and zinc are some of the elements currently under investigation for their possible relationship to heart disease.

The amount of any mineral that is taken up by the body from food depends on many factors. Phytic acid and dietary fibre both affect mineral absorption and are present in significant amounts in a wholefood diet. Phytic acid, found in nuts, wholegrain cereals and pulses, combines with essential minerals (calcium, iron, manganese and zinc) in food, rendering them unavailable for absorption into the bloodstream. The body, however, appears to adapt to phytic acid and eventually there is increased mineral absorption. It seems that there is an enzyme, secreted in digestive juices, which is able to degrade phytic acid. Phytic acid is also partially degraded by enzymes in yeast during the proving of bread, and in pulses when they are soaked in water.

Dietary fibre from plants may also bind minerals, but absorption is increased slowly after a change to a high-fibre diet. Poor mineral absorption due to phytic acid and fibre is only significant when a very restricted diet is eaten. Furthermore, since a diet high in wholegrain cereals and vegetables increases the intake of minerals, they will limit any deleterious effects on mineral status of the phytate or fibre associated with these foods.

### Calcium

Calcium is the most abundant mineral in the body. The bones – the supportive framework of the body – are hardened with calcium absorbed from food during growth. It is also necessary for tooth formation, for the normal activity of nerves and muscles, the activity of several enzymes, and for clotting of the blood.

Milk, most cheeses and yoghurt are the richest sources of calcium. There is virtually no calcium in butter, double cream or cream cheese, however. Products made from white flour, which is fortified, are also good sources. Some dark green vegetables, like watercress, are good sources, but spinach contains oxalic acid which renders most of the calcium unabsorbable. Wholegrain cereals, nuts and pulses, and eggs are moderate sources. Poor sources include meat, fruit and fish (except fish with very small bones which are usually eaten). Hard water may add significant quantities of calcium to the diet, but soft water contains little.

Too little calcium in the bodies of young children results in stunted growth and rickets (where the leg bones are deformed). In Britain, rickets is unlikely to be caused by low levels of calcium in the diet, for the body can normally adapt to these; the primary deficiency is of vitamin D, which promotes absorption of calcium from the small intestine. Only 20–30 per cent of the calcium in the diet is normally absorbed and the remainder is lost in the faeces.

Without adequate amounts of vitamin D, however, there is little or no absorption.

For the majority of people, a high calcium diet is not harmful because intakes in excess of needs do not pass into the bloodstream. By contrast, vitamin D is toxic when taken in excess: too much calcium is absorbed from food and deposited in blood vessels, sometimes with fatal results.

HOW MUCH CALCIUM DO CHILDREN NEED?

After birth, a baby's calcium needs are met by either breast milk or infant formula. Pre-school children need to obtain 600 mg calcium daily. The amount of calcium present in 100 g (3½ oz) portions of some basic foods rich in this mineral is as follows:

```
100 g (3½ oz) Cheddar cheese        800 mg
100 g (3½ oz) sardines (canned)      550 mg
100 ml (⅙ pt) milk      120 mg
2 eggs (size 4)      52 mg
4 tablespoons winter cabbage (boiled for 15 minutes)      38 mg
2½ medium slices wholemeal bread      23 mg
```

## Phosphorus

Phosphorus is the second most abundant mineral in the body and, in the form of various phosphates, has a wide variety of essential functions.

It is a vital constituent of all cells and, with calcium, provides the strength for the bones and teeth. Phosphates play an essential role in the liberation and utilization of energy from food. They are also constituents of nucleic acids and some fats, proteins and carbohydrates, and must be combined with some B vitamins in the body before the latter can be active.

All foods, with the exception of fats and sugar, contain some phosphorus, but sources of calcium and protein (milk, cheese, meat, fish and eggs) are richest. Cereals, nuts and pulses contain substantial amounts of phosphorus. Phosphorus is also added to food by manufacturers, in the form of food additives (for example as polyphosphates, raising agents, and phosphoric acid in some soft drinks).

HOW MUCH PHOSPHORUS DO CHILDREN NEED?

It is thought that children over one year old require similar amounts of phosphorus daily to calcium. Because phosphorus is present in nearly all foods, deficiency is unknown in children eating a normal diet. Absorption of phosphorus may be impaired, however, by the prolonged use of antacids.

High intakes of phosphorus in the first few days after birth may produce low levels of calcium in the blood, and muscular spasms (tetany). This can result from the use of fresh cows' milk, which has a high ratio of phosphorus to calcium compared with human milk, and in which the calcium may combine with the fat present and be poorly absorbed. Artificial formulas therefore have a reduced phosphorus content. Excessive daily intake of phosphate in older children may result in the premature cessation of bone growth and a subsequent reduction in adult height.

## Sulphur

Sulphur is mainly present as part of certain amino acids – the building blocks of protein. Nearly all dietary sulphur is derived from protein.

Sulphur dioxide has been added to food for many years as a permitted preservative. Its safety is under investigation, however. When food is stored for a long time, sulphur dioxide may react with fats to form toxic substances. It has also been found to cause genetic damage to some bacteria at very high dosages.

## Potassium

Potassium is present largely in the fluids within the body cells where its concentration is carefully controlled. Potassium has a complementary action with sodium in the functioning of cells. Studies in children indicate that diets rich in potassium can limit the high blood pressure which may develop when salt intake is high. Since potassium is frequently found together with sodium in foods, those foods which have a high ratio of potassium to sodium may protect against the development of high blood pressure.

Nearly all foods – except sugar and fats – contain potassium. Rich sources are yeast and meat extracts, wheatgerm and dried fruits. Nuts, meat, fish, wholemeal bread, potatoes, vegetables and fruits, are also good sources. White bread, milk and eggs are poor sources. Most of the potassium in the diet comes from vegetables, meat and milk. Fruit and fruit juices are noteworthy as being much richer in potassium than sodium. Like sodium, most of the potassium in the diet is absorbed.

The refining, industrial processing, and cooking of foods tends to leach out the potassium. In the home, however, potassium can be recovered in cooking water. Alternatively, foods may be baked or fried without loss of potassium.

HOW MUCH POTASSIUM DO CHILDREN NEED?

There is no recommended intake for potassium. Almost all foods contain potassium, so it is easy for a child to obtain adequate amounts.

Potassium deficiency is rare in healthy children and usually occurs only when there are increased losses from the body, for example in chronic diarrhoea or vomiting. Severe deficiency ultimately results in heart attacks. In health, a high potassium diet is not harmful – the excess is eliminated by the kidneys.

## Sodium and chlorine

All body fluids contain salt (sodium chloride). These elements are involved in maintaining the water balance of the body, and sodium is also essential for muscle and nerve activity. The amount of sodium in the body is kept constant; in temperate climates the quantity of sodium gained from natural foods is balanced by equivalent losses in the urine. This balance can be upset by excessive losses of salt in perspiration, which sometimes occurs for the first week or two in a hot environment. The body then acclimatizes so as to conserve essential salts. In Britain, adding salt to food is only necessary for people (e.g. miners) whose body temperature alternates rapidly between very hot and cold.

Some foods – meat, fish, eggs and milk – naturally contain small amounts of sodium. Others – flour, unsalted butter, cream, oil, fresh vegetables, and unsalted nuts – contain virtually none. Sodium is also found in many chemical additives. These include monosodium glutamate (found in many convenience foods), bicarbonate of soda (baking powder), sodium benzoate, sodium citrate, sodium nitrate and nitrite (present in bacon, ham, etc.). Foods to which salt is added include all cured meats and fish, sausages, pickles, sauces, most canned foods, salted snacks, most breakfast cereals, bread, crisps, olives, roasted nuts, cheese, salted butter, margarine, yeast and meat extracts, tinned and packet soups – in fact, most processed foods.

The amount of salt that babies need is provided by breast milk or infant formula. Any more than this, for example in household cows' milk, could be harmful, as an infant's immature kidneys require more water to eliminate excess sodium than adult kidneys. The sodium-excreting capacity of the kidney does not reach adult levels until the second year.

After weaning, children obtain enough salt for their needs from natural foods (meat, milk), without salt being added to food during cooking or at the table. Salt deficiency only occurs if the child is suffering from diarrhoea and vomiting, or if he has certain hormonal or kidney disorders.

In Western societies, salt is consumed far in excess of body needs. This is potentially harmful, since it can lead to high blood pressure in susceptible individuals – between 10 and 20 per cent of the population. Animal studies have shown that high intakes of salt during early life predispose towards high blood pressure in adult-hood. Once high blood pressure has developed, secondary processes act and salt restriction is of minor benefit unless carried to extremes. If salt restriction is therefore to play a significant role in reducing the incidence of high blood pressure, it must take place throughout life and particularly during childhood. High intakes of salt in the diet have been shown to be associated with stomach cancer.

## Magnesium

Most of the magnesium in the body is present in the bones; but it is also an essential constituent of all cells and is necessary for the functioning of some of the enzymes which are involved in energy utilization.

Magnesium is contained in many foods. Wholegrain cereals, nuts and spinach are good sources (particularly bran and wheatgerm products), but oxalic acid in spinach is known to interfere with absorption. Moderate sources include meat, cheese, fish, bananas, blackberries, peas, fried potatoes and raisins. White sugar, fats, some convenience foods and soft drinks contain virtually none. Less than half is normally absorbed and, unlike calcium, its absorption is unaffected by vitamin D.

Magnesium is little affected by processing and cooking, apart from losses in milling (wholemeal flour contains at least four times more than white), and leaching into cooking water. Up to two thirds can be lost when vegetables are boiled, but is recovered if the liquor is used for gravy or sauce. Fried, baked and grilled foods retain all their magnesium.

## HOW MUCH MAGNESIUM DO CHILDREN NEED?

Provided a child is eating a mixed diet and has no underlying disease, he will be obtaining adequate supplies of magnesium. Deficiency is rare and results from excessive losses in diarrhoea or poor absorption (for instance, coeliac disease) rather than from low intake. Excess magnesium is not toxic because it is not absorbed into the bloodstream. Magnesium salts (Epsom salts), however, are potentially harmful and should not be given to young children.

## Iron

Iron is needed for red blood cell formation. It is part of haemoglobin, the red pigment of red blood cells, which transports oxygen from the lungs to all parts of the body. Iron is also present in the muscle protein and is stored to some extent in organs such as the liver.

Only a small proportion of iron in food is absorbed into the bloodstream during digestion. Absorption is increased, however, when the body's stores are depleted and when needs are greatest. The iron in some foods is better retained than in others. Iron is most readily absorbed from meat, including offal (up to 25 per cent). Only 5 per cent or less of other forms of iron, such as those in eggs and vegetables, or added to flour, is absorbed; the exact amount depends on other factors in the diet. Absorption from those foods is increased by foods rich in vitamin C, such as orange juice, and by meat, whereas tea decreases iron absorption.

The richest sources of well-absorbed iron are black sausage, liver, kidneys and red meat. Other meat, fatty fish (sardines) and soya beans are also good sources. White fish contains comparatively little. Some vegetable foods – wholegrain cereals, other pulses, nuts, dark green vegetables – and eggs are apparently good sources, but other constituents (like phytic acid) render most of the iron in these foods unavailable for absorption. Thus, although spinach contains similar amounts of iron to beef, about ten times the weight of spinach would have to be eaten for the equivalent amount of iron to be absorbed.

Poor sources of iron are sugar, fats, milk, cheese, yoghurt and fresh fruit. Like other minerals, iron leaches out of food into cooking water but can be recovered if the liquid is used for soup, sauces or gravy.

HOW MUCH IRON DO CHILDREN NEED?

When available, iron is transferred from the mother in the last stages of pregnancy. This store tides the normal-weight, full-term infant over the first six months after birth. Premature and full-term infants of low birth weight, however, have a small blood volume and hence smaller stores of iron to tide them through the milk-feeding period. Although breast milk provides little iron, it is better absorbed than that from fresh cows' milk, and iron and vitamin C is added to certain brands of powdered baby milk. Iron-rich foods – meat – should always be introduced at weaning (between four and six months).

Babies need about 6 mg of iron daily, rising to 8 mg for pre-school children. These figures allow for its limited absorption. The amount of iron present in 100 g (3½ oz) portions of some basic foods rich in this mineral is as follows:

> 100 ml (⅙ pt) milk      0.05 mg
> 2 eggs (size 4)      2.0 mg
> 1 large slice fried lamb's liver      10.0 mg
> 3 heaped tablespoons grilled cod      0.4 mg
> 2½ medium slices wholemeal bread      2.5 mg
> Winter cabbage (boiled for 15 minutes)      0.4 mg

White bread and some weaning foods and breakfast cereals also contain added iron.

Lack of iron in the diet results in anaemia. It is one of the commonest nutritional disorders, affecting children in the developed countries as well as in the Third World. Anaemia may occur in infancy if stores of iron are inadequate at birth, if exclusive breast-feeding is prolonged for longer than about six months, or if iron-rich weaning foods are not given. Older children risk anaemia if food provides insufficient iron to replace the body's losses and iron stores become depleted. Children who are allowed to drink milk which is poor in iron, at the expense of eating iron-rich foods, are particularly vulnerable. Children suffering from iron deficiency anaemia will look pale in the face and the inside of the eyelids will be a pale colourless membrane instead of a healthy pink colour. They will be tired, lack stamina and show an inability to concentrate. Many also have a reduced resistance to infection and stunted growth.

Iron taken in excess is toxic and may be fatal.

### Fluorine

Fluorine is a trace element. It is found in bones and teeth. In food and drink it is usually called fluoride. There is as yet no direct evidence, however, to prove that it is essential for humans. It appears to harden teeth enamel by combining with calcium phosphate, and it has been shown that traces of fluoride are beneficial in protecting teeth against decay, the protective effect being most noticeable in children under eight years of age.

Drinking water is the main source of fluoride in the diet but the natural content is variable and is often below the optimum level of 1 mg/litre (one part per million). The only other important source of fluoride in the diet is tea and seafood, especially fish in which the bones are eaten. Too much fluoride in the diet results in mottling of the teeth.

### Zinc

Zinc is a trace element. It is necessary for growth, sexual maturity, wound healing, and taste and flavour perception.

Animal foods – milk, meat and fish – are the best sources, and animal protein may enhance its absorption into the bloodstream. It appears to be less well digested from plant foods and vegetarians may require more zinc than meat eaters.

Severe deficiency is unlikely in Britain, but mild deficiency, affecting taste and smell – which would impair appetite and growth – is now believed to be common in Britain. In animals, excess copper or cadmium can displace zinc in the body, but it is not known if deficiency can also occur in this way in man. Excess zinc can cause copper deficiency and very large intakes are toxic.

### Copper

Copper – a trace element – is necessary for growth in children and is part of many enzymes, including those needed for the formation of blood and bone.

Liver is the outstanding source of copper. Unrefined cereals (like wholemeal bread) supply more copper than refined ones (like white bread). Milk, most dairy products and eggs are poor sources. Some infant formulas are fortified with copper.

Adults are unlikely to be deficient in copper unless they are suffering from diseases causing malabsorption of nutrients from food. Infants who are dependent on one food – milk – which is poor in copper, for the first few months after birth, are more at risk. Normally, copper is transferred from the mother towards the end of pregnancy and held in store in the liver. This store tides the infant over until weaning. Breast milk contains more copper than cows' milk, and premature babies who lack adequate copper stores and are not breast-fed may suffer from copper deficiency. Symptoms include failure to thrive, diarrhoea, anaemia and bone fractures. Replacement of copper in the diet cures the condition.

Animal experiments suggest that other trace elements – cadmium, lead and zinc, may interfere with the absorption of copper from food. The high ratio of zinc to copper in cows' milk compared with breast milk may be a contributory factor in copper deficiency in infancy. Copper is toxic in excess.

## Iodine

Iodine – a trace element – is needed by the thyroid gland for synthesis of thyroid hormones which regulate many diverse and important body processes.

The most reliable source of iodine is seafood; the amount in animal foods depends on the level in the animal's diet, and the amount in vegetable and cereal foods depends on the level in the soil.

During infancy and childhood, increased amounts of iodine may be required to ensure adequate supplies of thyroid hormones during growth. These needs are unlikely to be met in most areas in Britain unless one or two sea fish meals are eaten each week, or fish-liver oils are given.

Lack of iodine in the diet results in goitre – an enlargement of the thyroid gland. It is endemic where the soil content of iodine is low, as in Derbyshire, the Cotswolds and the Mendips. In some areas, goitre is found despite a moderate iodine water content, and genetic and other factors are thought to be involved. Some green vegetables, for instance cabbage and mustard greens, contain goitre-inducing substances which have been shown to cause goitre in animals. In Britain, humans probably consume too little of these foods to be affected.

Iodine is toxic in excess. It causes the thyroid gland to become overactive and results in the disease thyrotoxicosis.

### Manganese

Manganese – a trace element – is associated with several enzymes. Tea, wholegrain cereals and nuts are rich sources. Some green vegetables (like spinach) are good sources. Refined cereals, meat, fish, eggs, fats, fruit, white sugar, milk and cheese are comparatively poor.

In animals, synthetic diets deficient in manganese cause infertility, and defects in bones and the nervous system. Manganese is toxic in excess.

### Chromium

Chromium – a trace element – is involved in the utilization of glucose. Diets high in fats, refined starches and sugar contain less chromium than those including plenty of fresh vegetables and wholegrain cereals. Large amounts of chromium may be lost during cooking and processing.

Needs for chromium are increased when the diet is excessively high in sugar or starch. Since refined starches and sugars are poor sources of chromium, even moderate intakes may cause a gradual depletion of body stores, resulting in mild deficiency in middle or old age. Symptoms occurring in animals fed chromium-deficient diets are raised blood cholesterol, increased evidence of atherosclerosis and decreased lifespan. The possible preventative effects of chromium in heart disease – in view of suspected large losses in food processing – are under investigation. Chromium is toxic in excess.

### Cobalt

Cobalt occurs in its free form in plants, but it is thought to be utilized by man only as part of the essential vitamin $B_{12}$ supplied in animal foods. Like other trace elements, cobalt is toxic in excess.

### HEALTHFUL DIET

In the affluent West, a healthful diet is one which not only prevents deficiency diseases and sustains a healthy life, but also contains all the essential nutrients in the proportions necessary to prevent Western diseases. One way of finding out what constitutes a healthy diet is to investigate the dietary habits of the most stable and healthy population groups in the world.

The bulk of these adult diets consists of wholegrains (rice, wheat, maize, etc.). Pulses (beans, peas and lentils) complement the grains and are eaten in approximately half the quantity. These two together provide the ideal proportions of the essential amino acids and form a good-quality protein (see p. 22). This grain/pulse combination is the basis of the meal and is given flavour and vitality by the addition of vegetables. These are usually eaten in larger amounts than the pulses but in smaller amounts than the grains. Green vegetables are most valued because of their higher content of vitamins, minerals and protein compared with most other vegetables.

In addition to the basic trio of grains, pulses and vegetables, most traditional diets contain varying quantities of a fourth group of foods which includes dairy produce, meat, eggs, fish and poultry. All the foods in this group contain vitamin $B_{12}$, whereas foods in the other three groups do not. This vitamin is necessary to prevent anaemia but is only needed in tiny amounts. A small daily serving of raw foods constitutes the fifth group. This may be fruit or raw vegetables.

Modern urban diets show a marked contrast to the traditional one, in that the most popular food items come from the supermarket rather than the garden. The typical British menu depends for its appeal on meat, salt, sugar, fat and artificial additives. These liven up the taste of refined foods which would otherwise be bland.

Modern eating habits, namely overconsumption of convenience foods, tend to reduce the intake of vitamins, minerals, essential amino acids, essential fatty acids and fibre. By contrast, there is often an excess of total calories, fat, refined sugar and salt. As a result, the diet either contains the correct number of calories but lacks essential nutrients, or it contains sufficient nutrients but too many calories.

Modern diets usually contain large amounts of expensive animal foods. These replace the vitamins and minerals lost when carbohydrates are refined, and deficiency diseases are rare. Although this diet may supply the recommended intake for all the known nutrients, it possibly contains too little of the lesser-known ones and predisposes towards such Western diseases as high blood pressure, heart disease, certain cancers, diabetes, obesity and tooth decay.

Breast milk or adequate infant formula provides sufficient nutrients for babies up to the age of six months and milk remains a very important part of the diet for the rest of the first year. After six months, however, milk can no longer supply enough of all the nutrients a child requires, and mixed feeding is necessary to give correct balance and quantity. Since a baby will not yet have acquired a taste for highly refined foods, it is possible to wean him on to a diet which bears more resemblance to a traditional one rather than a 'modern' one, without the objections one might get from an older child!

The grain requirements of such a diet can be met by the use of whole grains such as wheat, rice, maize, barley, oats, millet and rye. Alternatively, they can be taken as bread, pasta or flour. A variety of dried pulses can be found in health food shops, supermarkets or grocery stores. Most of these need to be soaked for several hours before cooking. They may be used in soups and casseroles or, ideally, combined with grains (beans on toast) to provide excellent sources of protein.

Freshly cooked green or yellow vegetables should be served daily, preferably in combination with the grain and pulses. If the child refuses them, they should be mashed and combined with something he likes (e.g. potato). The raw part of the diet can be provided by fresh fruit until the child is old enough to digest salads (one to two years).

Meat, fish, eggs, soya bean curd (tofu) or dairy products should also be included at each meal, but large amounts are not needed if the diet includes the foods described above and 'empty' calories such as sugar are not eaten. Some fat-containing food is necessary at meal-times – milk, meat, fatty fish, butter, vegetable oils, etc. – since fat is rich in the energy a young child needs and is a carrier for fat-soluble vitamins. After weaning, whole milk should be drunk daily by those children able to tolerate it and the diet should be supplemented with a natural source of vitamins A and D (fish-liver oil).

### How many calories should children have?

A calorie is a measure of heat produced when some substance is burned or oxidized. For most people, carbohydrate is the major material which is burned to produce heat to supply the energy needed for the body's functioning. One gram of dietary carbohydrate produces 3.75 kcal (16 kJ). A gram of fat (which is designed for compact storage) produces 9 kcal (37 kJ). When burned for energy, a gram of protein produces 4 kcal (17 kJ) – if one is so unwise as to use it for this purpose. A person needs to obtain as many calories as he uses, but if he is overweight he should obtain a few less than he will use. The remainder will be supplied by the use of fat stores.

Counting the calories a child consumes is a waste of time. His caloric needs can most accurately be judged from the signals his body provides. As long as carbohydrate is accompanied by the other nutrients – protein, fat, vitamins, minerals, etc. – which are normally combined with it in nature, the taste buds and the sense of hunger become a reliable index of how much should be eaten. It is primarily when 'empty' calories – that is carbohydrates such as refined sugar and starch which have been separated from the other components of food – or large amounts of fat are eaten that the problems of excess caloric intake and associated obesity arise.

# 3

# FOOD PROCESSING

Many foods cannot be eaten in their natural state. The preparation process may be simple, such as peeling (oranges, etc.) or more complicated: wheat grains, which must be separated from the inedible parts of the plant before they are milled into flour, which in turn may need to be treated before being baked into bread. At each stage of preparation some of the nutrients will be discarded or destroyed, whether the process takes place in a factory or in the home. The loss of nutrients that occurs in the kitchen is frequently equal to, or greater than, those which occur in the factory. The nutrients may also be destroyed if the food has to be stored for long periods, particularly if the conditions are not ideal.

Whole or natural foods are considered to be those foods which have suffered from little, if any, processing. Whole grains, pulses, fresh fruit, vegetables, meat, fish and dairy produce are all wholefoods; so is wholemeal bread, whereas white bread is not. Wholefoods do not generally contain artificial preservatives, so they do not keep as long as refined foods.

Junk foods are highly refined foods which offer little towards building health. They often contain substantial amounts of fat, salt and sugar, in a form that cannot easily be recognized. Highly processed foods are more likely than wholefoods to cause problems to children suffering from an allergy due to an unknown allergen. This is because, with processed foods, it is more difficult to identify the ingredient responsible. Even when the allergen is known, it is not easy to find out whether or not a food contains the substance in question, since the labelling does not always make this clear. Malt, for example, is made from sprouted barley or wheat and is frequently used as a flavouring. Products containing either malt or 'flavouring' may therefore cause problems in a child allergic to wheat.

Junk foods include sweets, jams, jellies and desserts, fruit-flavoured drinks, imitation cream, refined breakfast cereals, hard margarine, processed cheeses, and all products made with white flour; also some cold meats, frankfurters and corned beef, because of the large amount of nitrates added to preserve them and produce their pink colour.

## PROCESSING IN THE HOME

Home cooking is a form of processing and is one of the principal ways in which the nutritional content of food is affected. Heat causes changes in food which in general make the flavour, palatability and digestibility of the raw product more acceptable, and may improve its keeping qualities. Heat may occasionally increase the availability of some nutrients (carotene in fruit and vegetables, for example). Nutrient losses are more common, however, being greatest at high temperatures, with long cooking times, or if an excessive amount of liquid is used. Vitamin C, for example, can be totally destroyed by heat. The losses of water-soluble vitamins and minerals may be reduced if meat drippings and cooking water are used for gravies, sauces and soups, instead of being discarded.

Home freezing may result in some loss of nutrients – when vegetables are blanched in water before freezing – but less than might otherwise result during storage. If the temperature of the freezer is kept below −18°C there is almost no further loss of nutritional value until the food is thawed. In general, differences between the nutrient content of cooked fresh foods and cooked frozen foods, as served on the plate, are small. If the frozen food has been cooked prior to freezing and then reheated, the difference will be much greater.

## PROCESSING IN THE FACTORY

Factory processing was originally intended to preserve food, so that the choice would be greater and independent of geographical area or the season of the year, and to reduce the time spent in preparing food in the home. Nowadays, processing is frequently used to create 'new' products, by the blending or mixing of different basic foods, and the addition of sugar, salt, flavourings, colour and preservatives.

The main commercial processes which cause loss of nutrients are blanching, heat processing, and drying or dehydration. The freezing process itself has little effect on nutritional value, and since the delay after harvesting is minimal, the nutrients present in the fresh foods are generally well retained. Blanching is a first step in the preservation of vegetables, whether by heat processing, freezing or dehydration. Small amounts of some minerals and water-soluble vitamins dissolve in the water or steam and are lost.

Heat processing in metal cans, and bottling in glass jars, reduces the amount of heat-sensitive vitamins, especially thiamin, folic acid and vitamin C. Dehydration (in air) has little effect on most nutrients excluding vitamin C. About half the vitamin C is retained, however, although all the thiamin will be destroyed, if sulphur dioxide (a preservative) is added. Prolonged sun-drying, for example during the manufacture of raisins, allows substantial changes to occur.

## THE PROCESSING OF BASIC FOODS

All foods, unless they are fresh and raw, such as fruit and salad vegetables, have been processed to some extent. The nutrient losses that will inevitably occur depend on the type and extent of the processing that the raw food undergoes.

### Milk

Cows' milk is the most complete of all foods (excluding human milk, of course!), containing nearly all the constituents of nutritional importance to man; it is, however, comparatively deficient in iron and vitamins C and D. Unlike other foods of animal origin, milk contains a significant amount of carbohydrate, in the form of lactose. In a mixed diet, milk is particularly valuable for its content of high-quality protein and easily assimilated calcium, and as a rich source of riboflavin. It also provides good nutritional value for money.

Most fresh liquid milk is pasteurized (heated to about 72°C for 15 seconds). Unpasteurized milk (raw milk) can be a carrier of dangerous micro-organisms. Pasteurization causes minimal destruction of nutrients, whereas leaving bottled milk on the doorstep (especially in the sun), or exposed to fluorescent lighting, will cause substantial losses of riboflavin and vitamins A and C.

There are many different types of fresh milk available. *Channel*

*Island milk (gold top)* contains the most fat (4.8 per cent). *Silver top* is less creamy and contains 3.8 per cent fat. *Red top* contains the same amount of fat as silver top, but it is homogenized, which means that the fat globules are broken up mechanically and distributed throughout the milk. *Semi-skimmed milk* contains half the amount of fat of red top; it may also be homogenized. The fat is completely removed from *skimmed milk*, together with the fat-soluble vitamins and most of the cholesterol, leaving all the protein and minerals. Babies under six months should never be given household cows' milk or skimmed milk. After weaning on to a mixed diet, children should drink pasteurized, full-fat milk (silver top is best).

Milk from several mammals other than the cow is used for food by humans, e.g. goats, sheep, reindeer. Goats' milk has a similar composition to cows' milk, but contains less folic acid. Anaemia has sometimes occurred in babies fed boiled goats' milk.

Milk may be preserved by sterilization (heating above boiling point), evaporation or drying (to remove water). The ultra-high temperature (UHT) treatment of milk (*longlife milk*) causes vitamin losses which are very similar to the losses which occur in pasteurization. More vitamins are lost during storage. *Sterilized milk* is subjected to a more drastic form of heat treatment, and correspondingly suffers from greater losses of vitamins.

*Evaporated milk* is prepared by the concentration of liquid milk at low temperatures, followed by sterilization. In general, nutrient losses are similar to those in sterilized milk. *Sweetened condensed milk* is prepared similarly, but since it contains added sugar, the processing temperature needed for an adequate storage life is lower. Nutrient losses are therefore also lower, and are generally similar to those that occur in pasteurization.

Vegetable oils can be added to dried skimmed milk to make *filled milks*. These are used for infant feeding. *'Non-dairy creamers'* are not milk products; they are a mixture of saturated fats, milk protein, emulsifiers and other additives, with hardly any nutritional value.

*Ice cream* is a mixture of milk, fat, sugar, emulsifiers, flavours and colour. Except for *dairy ice cream*, commercial varieties do not contain cream. The fat in ice cream is usually hardened vegetable oil, containing antioxidants. In dairy ice cream, all the fat must be from milk.

## Butter

Butter is a concentrated milk fat. It is 82 per cent fat and contains vitamins A, D and E, but virtually no calcium, protein or B vitamins. Butter contains cholesterol. The natural colour of butter is due to carotene (from grass), but colourings may be added to pale butter, especially in winter. Up to 2 per cent salt may be added as a flavour enhancer and preservative. Antioxidants may not legally be added to retail butter, but butter sold for manufacturing or catering purposes is permitted to contain them.

## Cheese

When rennet is added to warm milk which may or may not be soured first, the milk proteins coagulate, forming a firm curd. This is treated in various ways to make cheeses of different kinds. Most of the protein, fat, and vitamin A, and much of the calcium in milk remain in the curd, while a large part of the lactose and B vitamins are lost with the whey. All cheeses have salt added during the manufacturing process.

*Cheddar cheese*, made from whole milk, consists of approximately one third protein, one third fat and one third water. Like most other cheeses, it is a high-fat food. *Cottage cheese* is made from skimmed milk and therefore contains very little fat; *cream cheese* has a very high fat content. Hard cheeses are, in general, more nutritious than soft cheeses because they contain less moisture, but they usually contain more fat.

*Processed cheeses* are pasteurized to prevent over-ripening, treated with emulsifiers to prevent separation of the fat and packed into moisture-proof coverings. Hard cheese may contain a small number of additives and specified colours. Soft cheese may contain additional additives, including flavourings, and cheese spreads and processed cheese may also contain emulsifying salts and other colouring matter. All British cheeses except Cheddar, Cheshire-type cheeses and soft cheese may contain nitrite but French cheeses may not. The white moulds normally present on some soft cheeses should not be eaten, as they are usually un-hygienic, and may prove to be potential carcinogens.

## Yoghurt

Yoghurt is made by allowing milk containing lactic acid bacteria to ferment. These bacteria partially digest the lactose in the milk and by doing so make it easier for the human body to use. Some children who are unable to drink milk, due to lactose intolerance, are able to tolerate yoghurt, even though it contains lactose. Natural whole-milk yoghurt has a similar nutritional value to whole boiled milk. Low-fat and fat-free yoghurts are made from skimmed milk powder; they have a slightly higher carbohydrate and protein content, compared with whole-milk yoghurts, but lack the fat-soluble vitamins (unless they are fortified). All (except pasteurized) commercial yoghurts contain living lactic acid bacteria and can be used to make yoghurt at home.

Supermarket yoghurts may contain additives such as colour, flavour, preservatives, thickening and jelling substances, and emulsifiers, in addition to fruit, fruit juices and sugar or artificial sweetener. Some are fortified with vitamins A and D. Natural, unsweetened plain or fruit yoghurts are best for children, rather than those containing sugar and flavouring.

Many health-giving properties have been attributed to yoghurt. It has been claimed that yoghurt can combat harmful organisms in the intestine which commonly cause a range of stomach upsets, often as a result of antibiotic therapy. Recent scientific evidence has shown that yoghurt consumption tends to lower cholesterol levels in the blood.

### Margarine

Margarine is not a dairy product but a butter substitute made by homogenizing a mixture of oils – animal, vegetable and marine – with brine. It contains as much fat as butter. All margarine must contain vitamins A and D; also frequently added are skimmed milk, salt, flavours, colours, emulsifiers and antioxidants. Almost any edible oils can be used for margarine and for low-fat spread, since they can be 'hardened' artificially by saturation with hydrogen (hydrogenation).

Margarine is often advertised as being 'made from polyunsaturates', but a large proportion of the fat must be saturated or the margarine would be liquid like any other polyunsaturated oils, even in the refrigerator. Hard, baking margarines contain less than 20 per cent polyunsaturated fatty acids (PUFA). Soft margarines contain about 30 per cent of their fat as polyunsaturates, but only those advertised as 'high in polyunsaturates' have a PUFA content of about 50 per cent.

Once an oil has been chemically hardened, a new 'fat' has been created. Since such artificially hydrogenated fats are a recent addition to the diet of man, and since the human body has had little experience with them, it seems reasonable to wonder if it has the capacity to deal comfortably with this essentially synthetic food.

In a recent study of the incidence of heart disease and the consumption of hydrogenated fats, dramatic correlation between the two was shown. Where margarines and solid vegetable shortenings were used in significant quantities, the rate of heart and blood-vessel disease was always higher than where they were not. It seems increasingly likely that eating hard margarine accelerates the process which causes this disease. Hydrogenated fats are not only found in margarines – many snack foods, refined oils, fast and fried foods also contain them.

### Vegetable oils

Oils are present in most grains, vegetables and even fruits. While they are still an integral part of the whole food, they are apparently beneficial, assuming that the diet is reasonably balanced. Once the oil is removed from the plant, however, it seems to become susceptible to a whole host of destructive influences.

Most vegetable oils are prepared by a lengthy process, known as refining. The oil-bearing seeds, nuts or beans are ground, steamed and then mixed with chemicals which act as solvents. The mixture is heated to drive off the solvents, but solvent residues are sometimes left in very small quantities. These chemicals are petroleum-based, and even small amounts of petroleum-based solvent are toxic and have been shown to cause cancers.

The crude oil is treated with caustic soda, bleached and deodorized, which removes the lecithin, minerals and variable amounts of vitamin E (which helps to prevent rancidity). Refined oils would go rancid immediately if chemical retardants (antioxidants) were not added. Many oils are partly hydrogenated (artificially saturated) too, again to improve their keeping qualities. The result of refining is the light, odourless, clean-tasting oil found in supermarkets, and often called 'pure' vegetable oil.

Certain oils – safflower, sunflower, olive, groundnut (peanut) and coconut, etc. – can be extracted by a process called 'cold' pressing. Coconut oil is the cheapest but least recommended of these, as it is naturally highly saturated. Although the pressure itself will often generate heat, this temperature is mild compared to those reached in the processes for refining oil. The unrefined 'virgin oil' obtained will contain few impurities and will be of edible quality without further processing. It keeps naturally for up to six months (longer in a sealed container in a dark place).

Many vegetable oils, especially safflower, sunflower, soya, corn and groundnut, are high in the polyunsaturated fatty acids. It is these oils that contain the essential fatty acids that are needed for health. They lower the cholesterol in the blood. By contrast, vegetable oils which are partially saturated, either naturally (palm oil, coconut oil) or artificially (margarine) will raise the blood cholesterol and should therefore be avoided. Olive oil is a mono-unsaturated oil and does not affect blood cholesterol.

Unsaturated oils are much less stable than the saturated animal fats (butter and lard) or the saturated vegetable fats (coconut oil) and easily become rancid. When they become rancid, highly dangerous little particles called free radicals may fly off and cause cell damage. Free radicals are produced when the oil has been heated, used for frying or even just exposed to light; they damage tissues and may be carcinogenic. Polyunsaturated fats are, nevertheless, needed in the diet. The answer is not to cut out the polyunsaturates, but to use them wisely and sparingly.

Cold-pressed oils are healthiest. They contain the lecithin and vitamin E which protect against free radical damage. The refined (heated) oils will have had most of these natural antioxidants removed and they will contain chemical ones instead. The long-term effects on the body of these chemical antioxidants is unknown.

Oil should be stored in a cool, dark place and the less stable polyunsaturated oils – sunflower, corn, etc. – used only for salads, etc. For frying, unrefined olive oil is best, since it does not undergo the same deterioration on moderate heating as do other vegetable oils. Alternatively, a little butter may be used. If possible, fresh oil should be used each time frying takes place.

Cold-pressed oils are expensive and often difficult to obtain. As an alternative, it is better to use good-quality oil from a specific source (e.g. sunflower or corn oil) in preference to a blended 'vegetable' oil of uncertain origin.

## Sugar

White sugar (sucrose) is made by refining sugar cane or sugar beet. It is so highly refined that it takes 1 kg of sugar cane to make 150 g of sugar. It is a pure substance and provides energy (calories) but is devoid of nutrients. It is harmful to health. The over-consumption of sugar is a major cause of many Western diseases, including tooth decay, obesity, heart disease and diabetes.

Brown sugar – from sugar cane – is less highly refined sucrose, containing traces of other sugars and minerals, and owes its colour to the small quantity of molasses it contains. It is not very different from white sugar since it is more than 99 per cent sucrose, and the quantity of minerals and vitamins contributed by the molasses is negligible. Some manufacturers produce an imitation of it by simply adding a syrup, caramel, or molasses to pure white sugar.

Genuine brown sugars are always produced from cane in their country of origin, which will be clearly stated on the packet. It may be Barbados, for instance, or Guyana or Mauritius. If this information is not printed on the packet, or there is a list of ingredients, then it is the manufactured variety. It is a mistake to consider brown sugar to be a nutritious wholefood – its effect on the body is virtually the same as that of white sugar – and all refined sugars are best left out of a child's diet.

Most white sugar is sold as granulated sugar. Caster sugar has smaller crystals and the particle size of icing sugar is even smaller. Syrups are highly concentrated sugar solutions. They include treacles, golden syrup and molasses. These contain 20–30 per cent water in addition to sugar, and small quantities of other substances. Molasses is a concentrated residue and is a popular folk remedy for treatment of several diseases; there is, however, no scientific support for its use. Molasses contains significant quantities of minerals such as iron and calcium, and trace elements, for example zinc, copper and chromium. Environmental pollutants such as lead and pesticides are also concentrated in it. Blackstrap molasses is the final residue of the sugar cane, and in the East is considered inferior, the least wholesome of the products extracted from sugar cane.

## Cereals

Grains are the commonest source of starch in most parts of the world, supplying the greater part of the fuel that is burned by human beings. Throughout the world, there is a wide variety of grains cultivated, and each climate and culture has its favourite, be it rice, wheat, rye, millet, corn (maize), oats or barley.

A grain is a seed and is made up of three parts: the germ, the endosperm or starchy bulk of the grain, and the bran or tough outer covering that protects the grain. The germ contains vitamins, oils, proteins and iron. It is an especially important source of vitamin E. The endosperm is made up of starch granules, the walls of which are mostly protein. Bran contains minerals and vitamins as well as cellulose, which is indigestible by humans.

Wheat is grown in Britain and is the grain most frequently eaten in this country. It is normally ground into flour but is delicious eaten as a cooked whole grain, or roasted and cracked (*bulghur*).

Wheat flour has a high gluten content and can be made into bread. It can be milled to different extraction rates. In 100 per cent extraction flour (*wholemeal*), all the grain is used. The flour is dark because it contains the outer layers of the grain (the bran) and the germ which are rich in minerals, fibre and vitamins. *Wholemeal bread* contains 8–9 g dietary fibre/100 g bread. In 72 per cent extraction flour (*white flour*) 72 kg of flour is obtained from 100 kg of grain. Almost all the outer layers and the germ are removed, leaving only the inner part (endosperm). *White bread* contains 2–3 g dietary fibre/100 g bread. *Brown flour* may be an 85 per cent extraction flour (containing most of the germ and most of the dietary fibre) or it may be a blend of white flour with bran added. *Brown bread* contains 5–6 g dietary fibre/100 g bread. *Wheatgerm bread* (Hovis, VitBe) is a bread with at least 10 per cent added processed wheatgerm.

Only the old stone-grinding mills are able to produce genuine wholemeal flour. Modern roller milling machinery can only produce a 'wholemeal' flour by making white roller-milled flour and mixing it back with proportions of the bran and germ. A loaf baked from such a flour is usually of larger volume than that produced from a stone-ground flour and almost certainly loses a lot of flavour and some nutritional value.

The refining of flour drastically reduces the content and proportions of vitamins, minerals and protein, and white flour is nutritionally inferior to wholemeal flour. For this reason, iron and two B vitamins – thiamin and nicotinic acid – must legally be partially replaced in white flour. Calcium is also added by law to all flour except wholemeal. No added nutrients are permitted in wholemeal flour. In spite of fortification, white flour contains far less magnesium, chromium, potassium, copper and zinc than whole unrefined flour. Other nutrients removed from white flour are vitamin E, some protein, almost all the bran, and most of the B vitamins.

The removal of the fibre from the wheat grain is probably the most important consequence of flour refining as regards health. Lack of dietary fibre has been held responsible for such diseases as constipation, varicose veins, haemorrhoids (piles) and diverticulitis, and partly responsible for coronary disease, diabetes and peptic ulcer.

Not only is white flour nutritionally inferior to wholemeal, but it may contain chemical additives. No additives are permitted in wholemeal flour – unlike wholemeal bread – but eight bleaches and improvers are allowed in all other flours. It is not surprising, therefore, that some people who appear to be allergic to white bread can tolerate wholemeal bread.

Other products of wheat processing include semolina (which is obtained wholly from the endosperm and is therefore mainly starch), and macaroni, spaghetti and vermicelli, which are normally made from semolina. Wholewheat pastas are made from the whole grain and are highly recommended.

While wheat is the predominant grain of western Europe and North America, rice is the staple of most of the Far East. Wholegrain rice, like wholegrain wheat, retains all of the nutrients, including those which are concentrated in the outer layers and germ. Unlike wheat, which is still most often eaten with little refining except in industrially developed countries, the bulk of rice eaten in the world is polished (refined).

Polished rice (white rice) is produced by removing the outer layer (bran) from the whole grain (brown rice). The outer layer contains a large proportion of the minerals and vitamins, especially the B vitamins. The largest loss is of thiamin, and beriberi is not uncommonly seen in those who subsist almost exclusively on polished rice. Brown rice – high in fibre and nutrients – is nutritionally far superior to white rice. Brown rice flakes, ground rice or flour – available from wholefood shops – may be used as weaning foods in preference to white 'baby' rice.

Oats are also grown in England and have a similar nutrient content to wheat, except that they contain more fat and biotin. Only the husk is removed during processing, and oatmeal retains most of its fibre and all the nutrients present in the germ. Whole oats are called groats; jumbo oats have been rolled once, porridge oats (pinhead) have been rolled more than once and oatmeal is a flour made from oats.

Rye is also home-grown. The nutrients in rye are present in roughly the same amounts as in wheat. Rye bread does not contain as much gluten as wheat, so it is rather stodgy. Some rye bread is coloured with caramel. In Britain most rye is eaten as crispbread. Wholegrain rye, rye flakes and rye flour may be bought from health-food shops.

Barley is grown in great quantities in this country; it has a similar nutrient value to other cereals and contains most of its minerals in the outer layers. Hulled (Scotch or pot) barley retains all the nutrients in the grain, but pearl barley has the outer bran and germ removed and the majority of the thiamin has been lost. Barley water is made from pearl barley boiled in water – it contains 2 per cent starch but little else. Maltose – a sugar – is formed in sprouted barley or wheat. Malt extract has a pleasant taste, but is not nutritious.

The nutritional properties of maize or Indian corn differ slightly from other cereals. It is deficient in the B vitamin nicotinic acid. In the UK, maize is eaten either as corn-on-the-cob (a special variety of maize) or as a breakfast cereal (cornflakes). Milling and toasting of maize destroys most of the B vitamins and brand-named cornflakes usually have added vitamins although, unless specified on the packet, cheaper varieties (like supermarket brands) can be assumed to contain negligible amounts. Commercial cornflour, used in custards and blancmange, is virtually pure starch and is a source of 'empty' calories. Whole maize meal is simply ground from the whole grain and is extremely nutritious.

Sago, tapioca and arrowroot are similar to cornflour in that they contain little except starch, but they are not made from cereals. Sago is produced from the pith of the sago palm, tapioca from the cassava plant and arrowroot from the West Indian maranta.

Millet is one of the oldest grains known to man. It is used principally in Africa and China. Whole millet or millet flakes are available.

## FOOD ADDITIVES

In addition to the expected ingredients of made-up foods, there are other substances which may be added in small amounts to perform a special function in food. These are called 'food additives'. They fall into two broad categories: those which are added to prevent food spoilage (preservatives and antioxidants, etc.) and those which enhance texture, flavour or appearance of food (emulsifiers, flavouring, colouring, etc.).

Permitted food additives are thought to be safe for both short- and long-term use. Safety tests are, however, necessarily restricted to animals, and the interaction of foods and additives to form toxic compounds cannot always be predicted. The effect of an additive on human health, therefore, may be uncertain until it has been in use for many years. More insidious is the possibility that if several additives are present in one product, they may interact to form potentially toxic substances. Government safety tests relate only to the toxicity of individual additives and not to possible combinations.

### Preservatives and antioxidants

Sulphur dioxide (E220) is the most commonly used preservative. It is an effective sterilizer (kills bacteria) and is especially useful in fruits, fruit drinks and vegetables because it prevents browning and preserves vitamin C. It destroys thiamin, however, and is permitted in meat products (an important source of thiamin) only if they would otherwise be a dangerous source of food-poisoning bacteria. Sulphur dioxide is a potential mutagen (causes hereditary changes in germ cells) and it has been implicated in asthmatic conditions along with another common preservative, sodium benzoate (E211). Furthermore, sulphited foods (E220–E227) have been found to become toxic after long storage.

Sodium nitrite and nitrate (E250 and E251) are salt-like chemicals used to preserve cured meats, including bacon and ham, some cheeses (e.g. Edam and Gouda), and pickled meats such as corned beef, tongue and some sausages. Nitrates occur naturally in soil, water and some vegetables. They are produced in the body and are only poisonous in very large doses. Enzymes from bacteria in vegetables and the human digestive system can, however, convert nitrates to potentially harmful nitrites.

Nitrite formation is more likely when little acid is secreted in the stomach, for example in infancy. Nitrite combines with haemoglobin – the oxygen-carrying pigment in red blood cells – and prevents it from transporting oxygen. This can prove fatal to babies under three months of age, as their haemoglobin is particularly vulnerable. Nitrates may not be added to baby food, nor may water of high nitrate content be used.

Under certain circumstances nitrites in food may form carcinogenic nitrosamines, and dietary studies in humans show positive associations between stomach cancer and cured meats which contain nitrites, and also environmental nitrates (in water, soil, fertilizers, etc.). Vitamin C inhibits the formation of nitrosamines from nitrites, and treatment of bacon – which is one of the major sources of nitrosamines in the diet – with vitamin C now results in far lower levels being formed.

Added preservatives must be declared on the label of most prepacked foods. Exceptions include food in small packages, fresh fruit and vegetables which have not been peeled or cut into pieces, cheese, butter, milk and flavourings. Preservatives are permitted on the skins of citrus fruits and bananas to prevent mould and children should not be given citrus peel in marmalade, cakes, etc.

In addition to the permitted chemical preservatives, there are the 'natural preservatives'. Acetic acid (in vinegar) is used to pickle vegetables, and lactic acid (from bacteria) preserves sauerkraut and yoghurt. Sugar and salt are effective preservatives, so are alcohol, some spices (cloves) and smoke (smoked trout, salmon). There is less destruction of vitamins when acids, sugar and salt are added to canned foods.

Most natural fats and oils contain substances (natural antioxidants) which prevent rancidity; the best known of these is vitamin E. Such substances may be removed or destroyed in manufacturing processes, for example during the refining of oil. Artificial antioxidants – e.g. BHA (E320) and BHT (E321) – must then be added to the refined products in order to prevent rancidity. Although the use of antioxidants is restricted, they are present in any refined food in which fat, oil or butter is an ingredient. Examples are crisps, frozen fried foods, biscuits and cakes. Baby weaning foods, but not baby milks, are the exception; no ingredient containing antioxidants (other than vitamins C and E) is allowed to be used in their preparation. Antioxidants are thought to be safe (except for babies), but BHA and BHT accumulate in the body fat, and their consumption by young children should be strictly limited.

## Colouring agents

About forty-five colouring agents are permitted. They are allowed in any food, except raw or unprocessed meat, fish, fruit, vegetables, white bread, tea, coffee and milk. Brown and wholemeal bread may be coloured with caramel only, and butter and cheese with specific natural colours.

Many food colours are synthetic coal-tar dyes, but some are products of natural origin, such as caramel (from sugar) and beetroot red. Coal-tar dyes are preferred by the food industry – they are less likely to deteriorate and, being highly purified, very small quantities are required – but the harmlessness of some has been questioned.

Tartrazine (E102), is an orange-red colouring agent which is added to many foods and soft drinks. It may cause urticaria (hives or nettle rash), asthma, migraine, hyperactivity, and many other allergies in those children sensitive to it. Paradoxically, tartrazine is used to colour some drugs prescribed for allergic conditions.

## Flavouring agents

About three thousand flavouring agents are used by the food industry. They may enhance the flavour of food, replace losses in processing and flavour manufactured foods (e.g. jellies, instant puddings, margarine and soft drinks).

Most flavouring agents are synthetic, but foods, herbs and spices, essential oils and salts, sweeteners and monosodium glutamate (MSG) are also used. MSG (621) is much used because it brings out the flavour of the meat in stews, meat pies, and so on; hence it is an ingredient of many sauces and is commonly found in potato crisps, savoury snacks, etc. MSG is known to produce brain damage in newborn rats and large quantities may give rise to unpleasant symptoms in humans. It also contributes to the sodium content of the diet. It should never be given to babies.

Sugar (sucrose) is the traditional sweetener; it is a rich source of energy but predisposes towards most Western diseases. Artificial sweeteners usually contain no energy, are much sweeter than sugar and are cheaper. Of the artificial sweeteners, saccharin is the most used; it is four hundred times as sweet as sucrose and provides no energy (calories) – it is permitted in soft drinks. Saccharin has induced bladder tumours in animals at high dosage and is banned in some countries.

Aspartame (Canderel) is the newest sweetener to be permitted in Britain; it does not have the bitter aftertaste of saccharin, but like saccharin is of limited use because it breaks down when heated. Aspartame is nearly two hundred times sweeter than sugar; it is permitted in soft drinks, yoghurt and as a table-top sweetener. It is made up of two amino acids. Both are found in steak, for example, but one of them – phenylalanine – when taken in concentrated form and without the rest of the substance in which it occurs naturally, has been found to affect the neurotransmitters, which are the chemical messengers of the nervous system. Some people are now thought to be at risk from Aspartame. Children suffering from the inherited brain disorder, phenylketonuria (PKU), are particularly vulnerable. The safety of Aspartame for the rest of the population is also being questioned.

### Emulsifiers and stabilizing agents

Emulsifiers and stabilizing agents are used extensively in the food industry in foods like bread, cakes, biscuits, meringues, cooking fats, sweets, soft drinks, jams, sauces and instant puddings. They enable fats to be used more economically, allowing them to be emulsified with extra water and making these emulsions more stable.

### Mineral hydrocarbons

Mineral hydrocarbons (905) are products derived from mineral oils. They are only permitted for use in a small number of foods. Dried fruit, e.g. raisins, may contain mineral oils to keep the fruit moist. The regulations assume that dried fruit is to be washed before eating, yet this is often not stated. Mineral fats can be added to the skin of citrus fruit. They are an ingredient of chewing gum and can be used to coat sweets. Processed food may also be contaminated by mineral oil present on processing apparatus.

Mineral hydrocarbons are undesirable in food, since they interfere with the absorption of the fat-soluble vitamins A, D, E and K. Small amounts may be absorbed and deposited in the liver, thus becoming potential carcinogens.

## Miscellaneous food additives

Acids give a sour or tart taste. Some are compounds which occur in nature, such as citric, tartaric or malic acids, or lactic acid. They can also be products of industrial fermentation. Thickeners, including pectins, vegetable gum and gelatins, give food their uniform texture and desired consistency, as in ice cream. Polyphosphates (E450 (c)) are used to process meats, especially frozen poultry, and meat and fish products such as sausages, hamburgers, meat pies and fish-fingers. They increase the water content of the product. Phosphates are used in soft drinks and in the production of modified starches. An excessive daily intake of phosphate can lead to the premature cessation of bone growth in children, with a consequent significant reduction in adult height.

Micro-nutrients are sometimes added to restore losses during processing; vitamin C, for example, may be added to fruit drinks. White flour is fortified with minerals and vitamins.

# 4

# FOOD POLLUTION

These days, people are increasingly exposed to a variety of pollutants, particularly chemical pollutants, in air, food and water. They are also ingesting a multitude of drugs. Sources of chemicals in the diet include additives, pesticides, fertilizers and the waste products from modern industry. Many of these are coal-tar products or their derivatives, and other synthetic compounds completely foreign to man.

Most drugs and chemicals act by slowing down or accelerating one or more enzyme systems. Since many of these may act together, only time will tell the possible cumulative effects on the health of minute amounts of many different chemicals. These could well be serious. Foods, for example green potatoes and peanuts, may also contain potentially harmful natural poisons and moulds.

## AGRICULTURAL CHEMICALS

The very high yields of crops now obtainable are largely due to the use of chemical fertilizers. The result has been not only a reduction in the nutritional quality of foods produced and the gradual destruction of the topsoil and mineral reserves, but a dramatic increase in the amount of hidden toxins which are consumed. Plants grown on chemically fertilized soil are not as hardy and resistant to attack by insects or competition from weeds as those grown on healthy, humus-rich soils, so insecticides and herbicides are used to protect them. The benefits of high food production are obvious, but the price which has to be paid is beginning to prove economically non-viable and environmentally unacceptable.

## Pesticides

Insecticides, herbicides and fungicides may find their way into food before it is processed, during farming, transport and storage. Food now contains more pesticides than ever before. This is because the pests have become resistant to the chemicals used, and the pests' natural enemies have been destroyed. Large quantities of pesticides are now needed where once smaller amounts were adequate.

Most pesticides are acutely toxic in relatively large doses, and although they are assumed to be safe at present levels of intake, animal experiments suggest that some might cause mutation of cellular genetic material, induce cancer, or, at higher concentrations, damage the growing child in the womb. Nevertheless, it is felt by most of those involved in food production that the benefits of pesticides outweigh the risks; without their use at least a quarter of the food grown would be lost. Some farmers have recently started to campaign for a return to crop rotation and traditional farming methods. This may reduce the need for pesticides by increasing the natural resistance of plants to disease.

## Nitrates

Artificial fertilizers of high nitrogen content are increasingly being used on farms to increase the growth rate of crops and of pasture used for grazing. Rain washes nitrates out of the fields and into the subsoil. They enter streams and rivers and eventually accumulate in drinking water. They cannot be removed by normal treatment techniques.

Nitrates pass through food and water into the body, where they are converted to nitrites. Nitrite affects haemoglobin in the blood so that it is unable to carry the oxygen needed for respiration. Babies under twelve weeks have an immature type of haemoglobin and are therefore particularly sensitive to nitrite poisoning, which can be fatal. Nitrate levels may rise dramatically after the first heavy rains at the end of a prolonged dry period; at such times bottled water is to be recommended for the reconstitution of formula feeds.

In adults, the concern is over the formation of cancer-inducing (carcinogenic) nitrosamines from nitrites in the body. These have been linked with cancer of the stomach.

Vitamin C protects against the carcinogenic effects of nitrites, so foods rich in vitamin C such as citrus fruits are especially important for children. Even organically grown vegetables and fruit are not exempt from high levels of nitrate, because of widespread seepage into land.

## Antibiotics and hormones

Antibiotics are permitted only to treat or prevent infectious diseases in farm animals but are often incorporated into the foodstuffs of cattle, pigs and chickens because they promote growth. They have also been used in food preservation. In these ways food may become contaminated.

It is possible that people who have become allergic to antibiotics used to treat an infection may be allergic to beef, pork, poultry or eggs and milk from animals treated with these drugs. There is also a likelihood that the small amounts of antibiotic present in animal feeds and in food could result in the multiplication of resistant strains of bacteria. A subsequent infection would then not be so amenable to antibiotic treatment, as the patient may have developed a resistance to it.

Certain anabolic steroids are permitted as growth promoters in cattle. Hormone residues in beef are usually very small, but the regulations governing the use of these drugs may easily be flouted and significant residues may be present.

## RADIATION

Food can become contaminated with radioactive materials which enter the environment either as a result of nuclear explosions or accidents in nuclear power stations, or by contact with nuclear waste. Radiation is highly dangerous in that it can cause cancer, birth defects and the mutation of germ cells.

Both water and soil are contaminated with radioactivity, but as plants absorb relatively little from soil, the outer parts – in direct contact with rain – are the most radioactive. Thus the outer leaves of vegetables such as cabbage are more radioactive than the inner ones, and wholemeal flour is more radioactive than white – though less of it is absorbed into the body. In general, foods of animal origin are more dangerous to man than those of plant origin, because the radioactive material is mainly concentrated in milk and meat.

## TRACE ELEMENTS

Traces of several elements not thought to be essential for health enter the body from food, water and air. Most appear to be harmless at low levels but high intakes of some, such as lead, mercury, arsenic, cadmium and aluminium, are known to have toxic effects.

### Lead

As far as is known, lead has no essential role or beneficial effect on the tissues. Ever since lead was first mined and smelted, people have been at risk of absorbing toxic amounts from drinking water, food and air.

Excessive lead intakes cause anaemia and damage to the kidneys and nervous system, especially in children. Fortunately, such large intakes are now rare. Relatively common, however, is the absorption of small doses of lead over a long period of time, whose effect is cumulative. This may result in a whole range of behavioural and mental problems. Among apparently normal children, for example, those who have absorbed more lead tend, on average, to be clumsier, slower, lacking in concentration, or of lower intelligence. Hyperactivity, temper tantrums, mood changes, sleep disturbances and speech problems have also been linked with lead. The less lead a child absorbs, the better. By knowing where lead comes from, and by taking a few precautions, the amount of lead absorbed can be reduced.

Much of the lead that enters the body comes from food and water. Shellfish, in particular, have a natural tendency to accumulate lead and other toxic metals and should be avoided by children. Game which has been killed by shooting will be high in lead, due to the presence of lead shot, which sometimes disintegrates in the flesh. Canned food, especially meat and fruit, usually contains more lead than similar fresh foods, since lead is present in the solder used for sealing cans. Babies should never be given adult canned food. If they must have canned food, they should only be given infant canned foods. Pure tin solder is used for canning infant foods; as a result no more lead is found in these foods than that which is present in the raw materials from which they are made. The amount of adult canned food that older children are allowed should be strictly limited.

Present legislation allows lead to be burnt in petrol. Most of it comes out of the exhaust and enters the air or is deposited on land. The use of some fertilizers may also result in soil containing high lead levels. When it rains, lead may be splashed up from the soil on to the vegetables growing in it. Vegetables from allotments near busy roads, for example, have been found to contain very high lead levels and should be avoided. Fruit and vegetables displayed outside shops on main roads may also be coated with lead dust. It is a sensible precaution to scrub or peel fruit, and peel or remove outer leaves from vegetables.

Water may be a source of lead in the diet. Soft water can dissolve lead from water-supply pipes. In hard-water areas, however, this problem is unlikely. It is important to check that lead supply pipes are not present before installing a water softener. Water drawn from the hot tap may have a high lead content and is undesirable for cooking, drinking or filling a kettle. This is true even in houses without lead plumbing, since hot water is liable to leach lead from solder in copper tanks or piping.

Dust in towns may contain high lead levels owing to the volume of traffic. It can penetrate buildings to coat food or crockery, and can also be directly inhaled. Children transfer polluted dust from their sticky fingers into their mouths. They should be kept away from car exhausts and babies should not be left in pushchairs near heavy traffic. Children should be discouraged from playing in or near busy streets, and windows facing main roads should be kept closed. Food and crockery should be kept covered to prevent dust from settling on it and, most important, children should always wash their hands before meals.

One source of lead may be the home. Old paint may contain a lot of added lead – even some new paints are permitted to contain a small amount. When stripping old paint, children and food should be kept well away. The amount of lead permitted in modern British toys is now strictly controlled, but old or foreign toys may contain dangerously high levels, especially if they are made of metal, or painted.

Imperfectly glazed earthenware may also pose a lead hazard, especially if acid fruit juices are stored in it. Commercial pottery is lead-free, but some hand-made earthenware is not.

A good wholefood diet helps children to reject most of the lead they ingest. Deficiencies of calcium, phosphorus, iron and protein have long been known to increase lead absorption. Hard water reduces lead absorption.

## Mercury

Mercury is not known to have any essential role in the body and is toxic in excess. It damages the brain and nervous system irreversibly. Mercury is discharged into the sea as industrial waste and as a result of natural erosion of rocks, causing contamination of fish. In Britain, nearly all the fish landed is relatively unpolluted, unless it has been caught in estuaries receiving effluent from large chemical plants. Pike, tuna and shellfish contain more than other fish, and should be avoided by young children.

## MISCELLANEOUS FOOD POLLUTANTS

Smoke contains carcinogenic polycyclic hydrocarbons. They are deposited on smoked, burnt and barbecued food. Icelanders, who eat a lot of home-smoked foods, have one of the highest rates of stomach cancer in the world.

Perhaps the most insidious and dangerous natural poisons are produced by moulds. It has only recently been realized that some seemingly harmless mouldy foods contain carcinogens. One of the aflatoxins, produced by a mould grown on poorly stored peanuts and other foods, is a potent cause of liver cancer in animals and man. It is worthwhile to avoid all visibly mouldy food in the home. The US Food and Drug Administration advises throwing away all mouldy food; trimming it off is not a sufficient precaution because the 'roots' may penetrate into the food. Moulds are more likely to contaminate food grown and processed without pesticides, preservatives and chemical additives. For this reason, extra vigilance is required by people eating organically grown foods.

5

# DIET AND WESTERN DISEASES

Many of the more prevalent diseases in Western societies – the so-called 'Western' diseases – are linked to dietary habits. These diseases may either affect children, or have their origin in childhood but only become apparent in adult life. They include tooth decay, blood-vessel and heart disease, obesity, high blood pressure, constipation, some cancers and diabetes.

Western diseases have been present on a large scale from the beginning of the present century and on a smaller scale from long before that. They are a direct result of modern eating habits. Over many centuries the relatively simple life of primitive man and beast has gradually changed to a complex, artificial and chemicalized civilization. Fresh food from fertile soil or the sea has been widely replaced by refined, processed and preserved produce of very different nutritional quality. The most important change in the diet, however, is the substitution of refined carbohydrates (such as sugar and white flour), for unrefined carbohydrates found in fruit, vegetables and whole grains.

Raising a child on a diet of highly refined foods does not necessarily mean he will suffer from a stroke or heart attack in later life. There are people who, in spite of smoking sixty cigarettes a day, or being obese, live to a ripe old age thanks to their genetic make-up. The chances of developing a Western disease, however, will be greatly increased, life expectancy may be reduced and the quality of life will be poorer than it might otherwise have been.

## TOOTH DECAY

Tooth decay (dental caries) is a common childhood disease; it affects about 40 per cent of five-year-olds. It is initiated by acids produced by bacteria in the mouth from dietary carbohydrate. These acids may dissolve the tooth enamel; and once a cavity develops it remains, since the enamel has little or no capacity for regeneration. As well as breaking down sugars to acids, some bacteria cause plaque to be formed on the teeth from sugar. Plaque protects the bacteria from the cleansing action of the tongue and so promotes tooth decay, and gum disease, too, in later life.

For nearly a million years, tooth decay was virtually non-existent. Today it is absent only in a few surviving primitive races and in wild animals. Although dental caries has borne some relationship to the practice of cooking food, it is mainly associated with the progressive removal of fibre in the refining of carbohydrates such as flour and sugar.

The refining of sugar has occurred more recently than the refining of flour. It seems likely, therefore, that the slow rise in the incidence of tooth decay from the Bronze Age onwards was chiefly due to the refining of flour, but the much faster rise in recent times is due to the refining of sugar. Although the starch in flour is converted by bacterial fermentation into sugar, any sugar eaten as such is clearly more quickly fermentable into the final acids.

When flour is refined it becomes much stickier, owing to the removal of the bran. It adheres to the teeth more readily and fermentation into acids is increased. The stickiness of the flour also causes sugar eaten at the same time to bind to the teeth and increases fermentation even further. Sugar eaten on its own does not adhere to the teeth as it does when combined with flour, since it dissolves very easily.

The frequency of tooth decay is more closely related to the number of times starchy or sticky foods are eaten in a day than to their total quantity. Sugary foods are also more damaging if eaten between meals rather than taken with meals. It is therefore less harmful for a child to have one concentrated sweet-eating session at the end of a meal, followed by a good tooth brushing, than lots of small refined snacks. Sucrose is not the only sugar to cause tooth decay. Glucose (dextrose), fructose, maltose, malt extract, galactose and lactose also cause decay, as does honey.

Infants and very young children are frequently given the taste for unnaturally sweet food at an early age. Infant formulas may contain glucose or sucrose, which are much sweeter than lactose – the natural milk sugar. Commercial baby foods are also often sweetened. Children's teeth are more vulnerable to decay than permanent teeth and the use of bottles and dinky feeders filled with sugary drinks, highly-sweetened vitamin supplements (fruit syrups), or even unsweetened natural fruit juices is associated with a high incidence of tooth decay in young children. This habit is particularly harmful between meals, especially during the night. Only water or milk should ever be offered by bottle. Rusks should also be avoided – even the 'low-sugar' varieties contain more sugar gram for gram than jam doughnuts.

Almost all breakfast cereals contain sugar, and additional sugar is often added at the table. In addition to the foods which one expects to be sweetened, such as cakes, biscuits, puddings, soft drinks and snack foods, many other processed foods which are thought of as 'savoury' also contain added sugar. These include such unlikely foods as certain brands of baked beans, tomato ketchup, tinned spaghetti, soups and vegetables, frozen beefburgers, gravy browning, corned beef and tinned ravioli.

Some foods protect against tooth decay. Apples and carrots have a scouring action if they are eaten after a meal; this reduces plaque formation. Cheese and peanuts are also protective; they increase the flow of saliva and have an inhibiting effect on dental plaque.

Fluoride is a mineral present in the dentine and enamel of teeth. It protects against tooth decay in children, and in areas where there is insufficient fluoride in the drinking water there is an increased incidence of dental caries. While fluoridation of the drinking water is widely regarded as the most effective method of preventing tooth decay, its implementation has proved either extremely difficult or impossible. For this reason other ways of providing fluoride for individual use have been adopted: among these are fluoride supplementation of the diet (drops or tablets) and topical application to the teeth by means of mouth rinses and toothpastes.

Fluoride supplements for children are currently available for use in areas where the water supply is deficient in this mineral. Too great an intake of fluoride results in mottling of the teeth, so it is important that the recommended dose is not exceeded. Supplementation should not begin until a baby is six months old.

Mouth rinses are not suitable for use by young children since their ability to use these is limited. It has been suggested that they should be restricted to children over six years old. Almost all toothpastes now contain fluoride, which means that children who are on fluoride supplements may be getting too much fluoride, especially if they eat toothpaste, or too much toothpaste is put on the brush by parents. The total avoidance of fluoride toothpaste by children under five years old who are on fluoride supplements has already been recommended.

## BLOOD VESSEL AND HEART DISEASE

Blood vessel and heart disease has reached epidemic proportions in the United Kingdom, and has its origin in childhood when 'furring' of the arteries begins. The role of dietary factors has been the subject of much study and still remains contentious. There is no doubt, however, that they are diseases of prosperous nations, and are rare in the underdeveloped areas of the world.

Various risk factors have been associated with an increased frequency of blood vessel and heart disease. These include diseases such as high blood pressure, obesity and diabetes, and also cigarette smoking, lack of exercise and stress. Dietary factors include high intakes of fats, especially saturated fats (animal fats or hard margarine), refined carbohydrates such as white and brown sugar and white flour products, and salt.

Future research will no doubt show which foods specifically contribute to coronary heart disease and which ones prevent it. In the meantime, the bulk of research indicates that a diet as unrefined as possible, which is low in total fats and oils, and high in whole grains, dried beans and peas, onions, fresh vegetables and fruit, will diminish the risk of coronary heart disease.

## OBESITY

Obesity occurs when an excess of fat accumulates in the body. It arises only when the intake of food is greater than the physiological need. In affluent societies adult obesity is so common as to be regarded as normal. Nevertheless, it is a contributory factor to the shortening of life by diabetes, heart disease and many other conditions.

Obese babies suffer from more minor illnesses than the non-obese. Many of these children become obese adults, and established obesity in adults is characteristically difficult to treat. Although obesity often runs in families, it is less likely to be caused by genetic factors than by faulty eating habits passed on from one generation to the next. The prevention of obesity in babies or small children is one of the most important prophylactic public health measures, and can obviate years of unhappiness and dieting in adult life.

Obesity in infancy may be due to the tendency of mothers to over-concentrate dried milk feeds during reconstitution, the addition of cereals to bottle-feeds and the early introduction of solids. It may also relate to the mother's behaviour towards her bottle-fed child. Women who seek to justify their satisfaction with the maternal role are liable to overfeed their artificially fed infants and use the child's obesity as a measure of their success in child rearing. Obesity may also result from over-protection by an anxious mother who feeds her baby every time he cries. Other mothers may feed their babies excessively either as a substitute for the love which they are unable to give them, or to make up for the feeling that they themselves were not loved sufficiently by their own mothers.

The single primary cause of obesity in an otherwise healthy child is considered by some experts to be due to eating refined carbohydrates (sugar, white flour, etc.) rather than the over-consumption of calories. The refining process causes carbohydrates to become unnaturally concentrated, which makes it easy to eat too much of them. Overeating fibre-rich, unrefined, unconcentrated carbohydrates (whole grains, raw fruit, potatoes eaten in their skins, etc.) is more difficult. Any wild creature in its natural environment demonstrates that no matter how plentiful the food supply, it never overeats. No wild creature, in fact, is ever overweight. Furthermore, there is an absence of obesity in humans whenever they are living exclusively on natural, unrefined foods.

Dieting and exercise will reduce obesity, but as long as refined carbohydrates continue to be eaten, it will always exist. The point to remember is that, provided only natural unrefined foods are eaten, one can eat as much as one wants without getting fat, because the fibre in the natural foods satisfies the appetite, so there is no desire to overeat. It is easy to eat too much sugar – but not too many apples.

The danger to health of carbohydrate foods should be assessed not by the number of calories they contain, but simply by whether they are natural or refined. Care must be taken, however, in deciding whether a carbohydrate food is natural, even if it is unrefined. Honey, for example, would appear to be a natural food, but until comparatively recently in evolutionary terms it has rarely been available. Man's metabolism is therefore little more adapted to the consumption of honey, which contains very little other than sugar, than to sugar itself. For practical purposes, honey should be regarded as being as harmful as sugar.

Once a child has become obese, dieting is essential. But in order to be successful in the long term, a child's eating habits should be modified. This may be difficult, as it is usually a family problem, so that other members of the family will need to alter their eating habits as well. Unless a child is grossly overweight, the type of diet normally recommended consists of ample amounts of protein and vitamin-containing foods divided into three meals, with no snacks. Items made from sugar and white flour (most processed foods) are excluded from the diet and animal fat is reduced in amount. A favourite wholefood item can be allowed daily – a few sugar-free, carob-coated raisins or peanuts, or wholewheat crisps, etc. – as the child has to give up many other enjoyable items of food to succeed in losing weight. This type of diet allows a child to avoid real hunger and yet lose weight safely and steadily.

Sometimes a mother may experience a psychological block when faced with her obese child. She may accept the need for a diet but cannot 'deprive' her child by withholding food. She will probably have had problems in her own childhood involving separation, and may be compensating by overfeeding her child for the input she missed out on. Sweets, and indeed any food with high sugar content represent for her the sweetness and love that she feels she was denied. It would be as hard for her to hold back on love as it would be to cut out sugar. Mothers with this problem are often over-protective – a typical 'killing-by-kindness' syndrome.

In order to ensure successful long-term weight loss, certain items of food must be drastically reduced in quantity or completely excluded from the kitchen. Sugar and honey should not be used at all, except on rare occasions. For all the family, desserts, other than fruit or plain unsweetened yoghurt, can be reduced to once weekly as a special treat, as can cakes and biscuits. Wholegrain bread should replace white, and unsweetened wholegrain cereals such as Shredded Wheat, Puffed Wheat and sugar-free muesli should replace the sugared varieties. Food should be grilled rather than fried. Potatoes should be baked or boiled in their skins; when they are prepared in this way they are filling and provide additional fibre. Roast potatoes eaten once a week as a treat should be large and carefully drained of excess fat. Chips, sauté, or small roast potatoes usually take up enough fat to treble the number of calories they contain.

Fat children tend to eat more quickly than normal-weight children, taking larger mouthfuls and more frequent bites. A fat child should therefore be encouraged to eat slowly and put his utensils back on the plate between mouthfuls. Prevention is ultimately better than cure. Childhood obesity could virtually be eliminated if mothers of new-born babies were encouraged to breast-feed and not to overfeed bottle-fed babies, and after weaning to offer only natural, unrefined foods.

## HIGH BLOOD PRESSURE

High blood pressure (hypertension) is thought to affect between 10 and 20 per cent of adults in Britain. It greatly increases the risk of stroke, heart attack and kidney disease, and, like heart disease, it often has its origins in childhood. Dietary sodium (salt) and excess calorie intake are two environmental factors known to play an important role in the development of high blood pressure.

Until recently, there were several human societies in which the use of salt as a condiment was unknown. In all of these the incidence of high blood pressure has been reported to be virtually nil, with little or no age-related increase in blood pressure. In Western societies, the blood pressure of the population increases with age, and this progressive rise begins before children are ten years old.

Children appear to be particularly vulnerable to high salt intake. Experiments on rats suggest that an increased salt intake for a period in infancy may influence adult blood pressure. Most authorities now agree that life-long adherence to a natural unsalted diet protects against the development of high blood pressure. Most people are not sensitive to high salt intake and will not develop high blood pressure as a result, but it is difficult to recognize those that are vulnerable; it is therefore a sensible precaution for all children to limit their salt consumption.

Land animals have evolved and thrived on natural diets low in sodium. It was not until early civilization that it was discovered that salt in high concentrations could be used to preserve food, and man slowly adapted his taste for salt to levels of consumption hundreds of times greater than that needed for survival. Babies are not born with a natural taste for salt, and it is theoretically possible to prevent them from developing one by offering them low-salt foods, and not adding salt during cooking or at the table. There is no risk that healthy children will suffer from salt deficiency, since even such basic foods as bread and cheese contain added salt.

Mothers may inadvertently give children too much sodium by feeding them on processed foods, most of which are manufactured with the addition of salt and other sodium-containing additives such as monosodium glutamate and baking powder. Particular care should be taken to avoid very salty foods such as Marmite, Bovril, and cured meats, such as bacon. Even processed foods that are thought of as sweet, for example cake mixes and breakfast cereals, are also salty too. All-bran, Rice Krispies and cornflakes contain more salt than potato crisps.

The amount of potassium in the diet influences blood pressure. Diets rich in potassium have been found to limit the high blood pressure which develops on a high salt diet. In one particular region of Japan, the lower blood pressure of the inhabitants and a reduced death rate due to stroke compared with other regions of Japan which have similar salt intakes, have been attributed to the ingestion of quantities of potassium-rich apples.

The refining, industrial processing and cooking of foods tends to leach out potassium, and in the canning of fresh peas, for example, the ratio of potassium to sodium may fall five-hundred-fold. Children should eat plenty of potassium-rich foods such as fruit, vegetables and fresh fruit juice as protection against high blood pressure in later life.

Weight gain also leads to a rise in blood pressure, and there is increasing evidence that weight loss may reduce blood pressure independently of any change in salt intake.

## CONSTIPATION

Constipation is delay in passage of the faeces. If a child has discomfort in passing the stool and it is hard and dry, then he is constipated. Simple constipation is caused principally by the removal of dietary fibre (roughage) such as occurs during the manufacture of white flour and sugar. Fibre is largely unaffected by the digestive processes and its primary dietary function is to absorb liquid and bind waste material as it passes through the digestive system. Lack of dietary fibre is associated with many diseases, including coronary heart disease, gallstones, appendicitis, peptic ulcer, diabetes, obesity, haemorrhoids, varicose veins and bowel cancer. Extremely low incidences of these conditions are seen in native races which do not consume refined foods.

Babies run the risk of becoming constipated as soon as mixed feeding begins, since most popular weaning foods, including rusks and fruit juices, contain refined carbohydrates such as white rice, white flour, modified starch, cornflour and white or brown sugar. Unless the ingredients of proprietary baby foods actually specify wholemeal or brown rice (rather than flour or rice), for example, they should not be bought; neither should products containing sugar (sucrose, glucose, dextrose, malt, etc.).

Inadequate fluid intake may also result in constipation when weaning is initiated.

As a baby gets older, white bread, cakes and biscuits and refined breakfast cereals are best avoided. Instead he may have wholegrain alternatives such as wholemeal bread, brown pasta, brown rice and unsweetened wholegrain cereals. Brown bread is not wholemeal; it is made from brown flour with a fibre content intermediate between white and wholemeal flours, which can be produced by milling off 15 per cent of the wheat grain. Alternatively, it may be a blend of white flour with sufficient added bran to comply with the legal requirement. Wheatgerm breads like Hovis or VitBe are not wholemeal either, but are made with white or brown flour with at least 10 per cent added wheatgerm and possibly caramel for colour.

Bran must not be added to a young child's diet as a means of preventing constipation; it binds certain essential minerals and vitamins and prevents their absorption into the body.

White and brown sugar, honey, sweets, chocolates, soft drinks, sweetened fruit juices, and ice creams encourage fibre-related diseases. As a sweet alternative, raw or dried fruit may be offered. If constipation should occur then the amount of fluids the baby or child is having should be increased and natural laxatives such as stewed figs, prunes or fresh raspberries may be given. Laxative medicines should never be necessary.

## CANCER

Diet may influence the incidence and rate of growth of tumours in a community. At least 30 per cent of all cancers are now thought to be related to diet. There is much to suggest that the wide variation in incidence of cancer at various sites in the alimentary canal and in the liver may be due to carcinogenic (cancer-inducing) factors in the diet. Carcinogenic agents in foods may be natural substances, such as fat, or they may be chemicals deliberately added to food (colourings). In many instances exposure has to continue for a long period, sometimes up to twenty years, before a tumour develops. Food habits learnt during early childhood could therefore be responsible for a tumour which develops in adulthood. Although some people appear immune to many carcinogens, many discover, sometimes too late, that they are not.

Cancer of the stomach is one type of cancer which has conclusively been shown to be related to dietary factors. The preservatives sodium nitrite and nitrate (E250 and E251) have been implicated. These preservatives are commonly found in some cheeses (Edam and Gouda), bacon, ham, luncheon meat, corned beef and some sausages. These foods are frequently offered by well-meaning mothers to babies and children. By reading labels carefully and not eating the above-mentioned foods, nitrites can largely be avoided. It should be remembered, however, that foods containing bacon, for example, necessarily contain nitrite although this will not be listed on the ingredients. High intakes of salt and smoked food are also associated with stomach cancer.

Large amounts of fat in the diet may result in breast or colon cancers. Meat is unlikely to contain carcinogens but they might be formed – by burning – during roasting and grilling. Low intakes of dietary fibre lengthen the time that foods spend in contact with the gut and so increase the risk of bowel cancer.

The artificial sweetener, saccharin, has induced bladder cancer in animals when given in high dosage and is banned in some countries. Many soft drinks contain saccharin, especially the 'diet' or 'low-calorie' varieties. These are often popular because they are cheaper than the sugar-containing varieties. Smoked or barbecued food is also carcinogenic. Barbecued food is less carcinogenic if it is wrapped in aluminium foil before cooking. This helps to prevent the food being smoked and charred.

## DIABETES

Diabetes mellitus is a condition characterized by a raised sugar (glucose) concentration in the blood, due to a lack or reduced effectiveness of the pancreatic hormone, insulin. The disease is chronic and affects the breakdown of fat and protein. Diabetics have an increased risk of blood-vessel disease. In long-standing cases specific changes can occur in the eyes, feet, nerves and kidneys. Fortunately, diabetes is not common in childhood, but when it occurs it is relatively severe and always requires treatment with insulin.

Diabetes is virtually absent in primitive communities who live on unrefined carbohydrates, and is considered to be a disease of prosperous nations. Some experts feel that the cause of diabetes lies essentially in the consumption of refined carbohydrates – sugar and white flour – which imposes unnatural strains upon the pancreas, either through overeating, or speed of eating and absorption, or both. Indeed, studies have shown that diabetic children are above average height at the time they appear at the hospital with diabetes, and children with diabetes are heavier at one year than non-diabetic children. This may indicate the presence of eating disorders in children who subsequently develop diabetes.

Since the majority of cases of diabetes are thought to be due to the consumption of refined carbohydrates (especially sugar), and only indirectly through loss of fibre in the diet, it is possible to prevent it occurring or to arrest early diabetes by giving a child an unrefined diet. This means removing sugar and honey products from the diet and replacing them with raw or dried fruit. White bread, cakes, cereals, etc., should also be avoided and plenty of wholegrain products, pulses, fruit and vegetables offered instead.

# 6

# IN THE KITCHEN

New parents are often bewildered by the variety of equipment on the market for babies. This is particularly true of kitchenware. Some items are essential, while many others, although useful, can be dispensed with, and standard kitchen equipment used instead. More important for a baby's welfare is to have a scrupulously clean kitchen and adequate food storage facilities, and to avoid any contamination of foods or equipment with food-poisoning organisms.

The way in which a baby's meals are prepared and cooked is also of great importance, since nutrient losses which occur in the home are often greater than those that take place anywhere else along the food-processing chain.

## MEALTIME EQUIPMENT

Bottles, teats and bottle-sterilizing equipment are essential for those babies not being breast-fed. But a baby breast-fed on demand should need nothing for at least four months until solids are introduced and extra liquids are required. This liquid can be taken from a small cup as long as the baby is still getting all his milk from the breast.

After weaning has begun, a bib is useful to prevent food from soiling clothing. The traditional bib is made of cloth, is not very effective and normally needs to be laundered after every meal. Moulded plastic bibs are a boon. They are easily washed and dried and have the added advantage of having a 'tray' to catch food which misses the child's mouth. One bib is quite sufficient, and it may be used from about six months until the child is old enough to use a napkin (this can be any time between two and four years).

Some children object to wearing this type of bib. It is so labour-saving, however, that it is worth insisting that it is worn. This can best be done by routinely putting the bib on the baby before presenting him with his meal, so that if he wants his food he will soon come to accept the bib.

A high chair enables a baby to eat his food in safety without having to be held. A harness must be used to secure him – it is a long drop if he falls out! A high chair may be used from the time a baby can sit up well, unsupported, until he is able to sit safely on a chair and eat his meal at the table – about two years. Some mothers, however, find it convenient to keep their children in a high chair for longer.

A high chair is a good buy if it is likely to be used by more than one child. If a high chair is not purchased, a baby can always be held, or he can sit up at the table in a plastic box seat (from about nine months). This has straps to secure it to most chairs. These seats cost a fraction of the price of even a cheap high chair, but a child must never be left alone while he is using the seat.

A baby's first solid food is often puréed. A food processor, liquidizer or blender is not necessary, however, since the amount of food required may be prepared with less washing up and wastage, using a simple grater and knife and fork. Finely chopped food can be given at six months, or even earlier. In fact, if a baby is fed on a diet of puréed mush for too long, it may be difficult getting him to accept the family diet.

Plastic bowls, plates, spouted cups, spoons and forks are all useful and prevent crockery from being smashed. Especially good are bowls with rubber suction bases to fix them to the table or high chair. Washable place-mats are also practical.

## FOOD POISONING

A child's health depends not only on the nutritional value of the food he eats, but also on the unwanted substances he ingests with his food. These include environmental pollutants, agricultural chemicals and the bacteria and viruses which may enter food and cause food poisoning. By careful handling and storage of food at home and excellent kitchen and personal hygiene, the ingestion of these 'invisible' toxins can be greatly reduced.

Most chemicals which enter food cannot be completely removed before consumption, or easily be prevented from entering it. Washing-up liquid – a detergent – is one potential food pollutant which can be prevented from entering food, yet is frequently allowed to do so. It remains on eating utensils, and sometimes baby's feeding bottles, which are allowed to dry without being rinsed or wiped. It has been suggested that detergent damage could lead to chronic bowel disease. Until further research shows whether ingesting tiny amounts of detergent on a daily basis is harmful, it is a sensible precaution to rinse all washing-up with clean running water before leaving it to dry.

Chemicals which contaminate fruit and vegetables – pesticides and lead for example – may be partially removed if all produce is carefully washed or scrubbed and the skin, peel or outer leaves (cabbage, sprouts) removed and thrown away. Inevitably, by removing the skin of potatoes, apples, pears, etc., the integrity of the food will be disrupted and some dietary fibre, vitamins and minerals will be lost from a child's diet. On balance, the benefits of eating the wholefood are likely to outweigh the health risks of ingesting tiny amounts of contaminants which remain after produce has been scrubbed or scrupulously washed. Of course, if a particular fruit or vegetable is suspected of being heavily contaminated, it should be peeled or preferably totally avoided. If doubt remains whether fruit has been washed when outside the home, then it must always be peeled.

Grain stores, e.g. of wheat, are frequently treated with pesticides. All whole grains (wheat, rice, barley, etc.) must therefore be carefully washed before cooking. The best way to do this is to cover the grain with cold water, swirl it in the water, then drain. This should be repeated several times.

Improper storage is often the cause of food becoming contaminated. When a tin is opened, for instance, its contents should be immediately removed and treated as if they were fresh. Some cans are lined with lacquer which greatly reduces the erosion of tin by acid contents (fruit juices, etc.). Other foods do not cause erosion in unopened cans, but once in contact with the oxygen in air, tin is rapidly dissolved. The amount of lead which leaches out of the solder into food also increases sharply when the can is opened.

Mouldy foods – cheese, jams, etc. – may be potentially toxic and should be discarded. Experts in this field do not consider that it is a sufficient precaution to just trim it off, and throw away the mouldy bits, because the 'roots' may penetrate into the food. Wholefoods, especially those which have been organically grown, are particularly susceptible to moulds, since they are generally free from chemical preservatives. It is best to store them under refrigeration and eat them quickly.

It is very risky to refreeze frozen fish or meat after it has thawed, unless it is refrozen after cooking. Micro-organisms which are capable of causing serious food poisoning are not destroyed by freezing, and when food is thawed to room temperature it enters the temperature range most likely to encourage growth of bacteria, yeasts and moulds, all of which could be harmful. Each time food is defrosted and exposed to conditions favourable to this growth, the danger rises. Food which is defrosted while still wrapped, in the refrigerator, and still retains some ice crystals, is therefore infinitely safer to refreeze, than food which has been unwrapped and allowed to stand exposed in a warm kitchen for hours.

The dangers from disease-producing organisms in food far exceed those from natural poisons (moulds) or man-made chemicals (pesticides). All food contains some harmful bacteria, although it may be quite safe to eat. A lifetime of exposure to this hazard makes one partially immune. Babies have yet to build up this immunity and tainted food can seriously upset them.

Many disease-producing organisms are excreted in human faeces and some in urine. Infection may be spread by transfer of the organisms by flies, or the human hand, to foods or food utensils. Hands should always be washed after using the lavatory or handling a baby's nappies or potty, and before preparing food. Children should also always wash their hands after using the lavatory and before eating. Once they get into the habit, they will accept it as routine. Dirty towels can be a source of infection and can reinfect hands which have been carefully washed.

Apparently healthy cats and dogs may also harbour infection. Horse meat or kangaroo meat used as pet food is commonly heavily contaminated with salmonella and if such uncooked infected meat is fed to cats or dogs, the probability is that they, too, will become infected and act as a reservoir of food-poisoning organisms.

Leaving food uncovered for even a few minutes in hot weather can mean contamination by flies. The nose and mouth are other sources of infective organisms, and coughing and sneezing can infect uncovered food up to a distance of 6 m (20 ft). Utensils which have been in someone's mouth should never be used to serve or taste food which is to be stored as leftovers. Dirty handkerchiefs and infected wounds are also potent sources of infection.

Most disease-producing organisms, and toxins manufactured by them, are destroyed by heat, and food which is properly handled and cooked is usually safe. It is crucial to allow food to reach boiling point (100°C, 212°F) and to continue cooking for sufficient time (up to 30 minutes) to kill all the bacteria and toxins. During cooking, however, the heat may not penetrate the food sufficiently, particularly a large joint of meat or a chicken which has not completely thawed before cooking, and under-cooked foods are unsafe, especially for children.

Food may also be contaminated after cooking; meat, milk and eggs are excellent growth media for bacteria. Left-over food should always be covered and refrigerated as soon as it has cooled, and definitely within an hour and a half. Hot food should never be put directly into the refrigerator, as it will cause a rise in temperature in previously refrigerated food, thus promoting the growth of organisms. Reheating food is particularly risky. Leftovers should always be fully cooked the second time, not merely warmed.

Salmonella is the chief cause of food poisoning in Great Britain and it is resistant to many antibiotics. It frequently occurs when bacteria are transferred from raw to cooked meat and these should always be stored separately. The same chopping board or knife should not be used for raw and cooked meat. Even a fork used to prick sausages before cooking should be washed immediately after use, in case it has picked up any bacteria from the raw meat. While environmental health departments allow raw meat to be sold alongside unwrapped cooked meats, pies, cheese, bread, etc., in many butcher's shops, it is a wise precaution to avoid shopping for anything but uncooked meat at a butcher's.

The foods most often infected by salmonella are meat (particularly processed meat such as pies), poultry, eggs and egg-products, custard, cakes, trifles and artificial cream. Chickens or other animals fed infected feedstuffs pass on the bacteria when they are killed for human consumption. Bacteria can be carried on chicken skin, in the offal or inside the carcass, so chickens should be scalded with boiling water inside and out before cooking. The cavity should not be filled with stuffing as the temperature at the centre may not get high enough to kill all the bacteria. Foods which have been contaminated with salmonella are safe to eat provided that they are subsequently well cooked. At temperatures of at least 60°C (140°F) all such bacteria will be destroyed. At 100°C (212°F) – the boiling point of water – all bacteria will be killed in one to two minutes.

Other foods which are commonly affected by disease-producing organisms include: gravy, stews, cream, ice cream, fish, shellfish, rice and cornflour. Food poisoning may cause abdominal pain, fever, diarrhoea and vomiting. Symptoms occur up to seventy-two hours after ingesting the infected food and can last from six hours to eight days. While most cases of food poisoning in adults will not need medical intervention, medical help should always be sought where children are concerned. Babies suffering from 'gastroenteritis' usually need to be hospitalized since they run a serious risk of dehydration and even death.

The severe and often fatal form of food poisoning known as botulism is now very rare. It has occurred after eating canned and bottled meats and some vegetables, and smoked food. The food industry adds nitrite to cured and smoked meat as a preservative to prevent the development of the poison which causes botulism. There is a risk, however, from smoked trout, unless it is refrigerated. It has recently been suggested that a small proportion of cot deaths is due to infant botulism. Honey exposure has been linked to this condition and honey should not be fed to infants under one year of age.

Many worms have complicated life cycles in which they live as parasites in more than one host. Man may be infected by eating undercooked pork, beef and fish, and raw salads. Prevention involves cooking pork, beef and fish thoroughly and soaking salads (particularly watercress) in salty water to kill the worms, and then rinsing several times in clean water.

## COOKING METHODS

Owing to its greater digestibility and palatability, much of the child's diet consists of cooked food. The preparation and cooking of food usually results in the destruction of some nutrients, particularly vitamin C. It may, however, increase the availability of others. Carotene, for example, is present in fruit and vegetables and is converted to vitamin A in the body; whereas only 1 per cent is absorbed from carrots eaten raw, 30 per cent is absorbed from cooked ones. This is because carotene is held within cell walls made of undigestible cellulose and these are broken down during cooking.

## Food preparation

All food must be prepared to some extent before it is cooked. The more complex the preparation, the greater the destruction of vitamins and minerals will be.

The washing of food often results in substantial nutrient losses. Leaving food, especially fruit and vegetables, to soak in water will cause the water-soluble vitamins – B and C – and some elements to leach out of the food. To keep nutrient losses to a minimum, most food should be washed quickly under running water just before cooking.

Peeling, shredding, chopping, crushing and slicing result in some loss of nutrients – especially vitamin C – by increasing the surface area through which losses may occur, and by setting free nutrient-destroying enzymes. This loss can be reduced by preparing fruit or vegetables (e.g. fruit salad, coleslaw salad) immediately before eating or cooking.

## Boiling

Food cooked in water loses a considerable proportion of its water-soluble nutrients by leaching. Small pieces of food suffer greater nutrient losses than food cut into large pieces. This is because the surface area through which nutrients can escape will be larger, and the release of nutrient-destroying enzymes will be greater. Destruction of nutrients also increases with the volume of water used for cooking and the length of time for which food is boiled. There is a drastic loss of vitamin C, for example, when prolonged cooking times are used.

To boil food so that losses are kept to a minimum, food should be prepared immediately before cooking, only a small volume of water should be used, and food should be plunged into boiling water rather than cold so that the destructive enzymes are damaged. Overcooking must be avoided.

At the end of the cooking process, there should be little, if any, water left in the saucepan. Any liquid that remains must not be discarded but should be saved to make soup, etc. Food which is kept warm continues to lose nutrients, so it should always be eaten as soon as possible after cooking.

## Steaming

This method of cooking involves using the steam produced from boiling water. The contact between the food and water is less than in boiling and there is a smaller loss of water-soluble nutrients. As a longer cooking time is required, however, the amount of vitamin C which is decomposed by heat is increased. Cooking water should always be saved.

## Stewing

Stewing involves cooking food in hot water below boiling point. The changes which occur in stewing are therefore similar to those which take place during boiling, though they occur at a slower rate. One of the advantages of stewing over other methods is that it makes protein food more digestible and it has a tenderizing effect, so it is a particularly suitable method for cooking tough meat. The disadvantage of stewing is that it involves a considerable loss of nutrients into the cooking water. Juices from stewed food should therefore always be used for gravy, soups, etc.

## Roasting, grilling and frying

These cooking methods use higher temperatures than boiling, stewing or steaming since the heat used is dry rather than moist. All nutrients are affected to some extent by dry heat apart from the mineral salts (iron, magnesium, etc.) which are stable to heat.

Fats are fairly stable to moderate heating, but when they are heated to high temperatures they start to decompose. Carbohydrates are affected by dry heat and so are the heat-sensitive vitamins, notably vitamin C and thiamin. The nutritive value of protein is not significantly affected unless it is heated to a fairly high temperature, such as occurs during roasting.

Frying causes similar nutrient losses to those which occur during roasting. Losses due to frying are minimized if the fat is very hot when food is added to it. Once fat has been used for frying, it should be thrown away. Most fats when heated to a high temperature form substances which are considered by many experts to be harmful to health.

# 7

# SHOPPING

Increasingly sophisticated food technology has meant that it is becoming more and more difficult to know exactly what is being bought in the shops, since most highly processed foods bear confusing labels listing incomprehensible ingredients.

Health-food shops can be especially daunting. The shopper is confronted with row upon row of anonymous cellophane packets, containing strange grains, fruits, seeds and beans, with no explanation of what to do with them and often little assistance available. It is hardly surprising that heavily advertised and readily available convenience foods are often preferred.

## SHOPPING FOR FRESH FOODS

The best fresh produce may be found in specialist shops (greengrocers) or markets. It is here that one is likely to get both the most choice and helpful advice. If a greengrocer or market are not within easy reach, a large supermarket provides the best alternative as it is likely to have a rapid turnover of fresh, high-quality food.

### Vegetables and fruit

The golden rule is to purchase the freshest seasonal vegetables and fruit. These have the highest level of nutrients, especially if they are grown in rich organic soil. Most vegetables and fruit (provided that they are correctly prepared) can be eaten by babies over four months, and virtually all of them after one year. A wide range of produce used in the diet will reduce the chance of deficiency of essential nutrients.

Most vegetables can be described as tender or hardy. Both are best young and freshly picked, but freshness is especially important when choosing tender types. Tender vegetables include lettuce, spinach, leaf greens, runner beans, aubergines, tomatoes, mange-tout peas and courgettes. Once picked, they are cut off from their water supply and become exceedingly vulnerable due to lack of water reserves in the plant. Leafy varieties wilt fast, fruit-like vegetables turn limp and soggy, and beans and peas become starchy and tasteless.

Hardy vegetables are more resilient when picked and are not as easily digestible as the tender varieties; these include members of the cabbage family, onions, celery, leeks, potatoes, carrots, swedes, turnips and parsnips. Most of these require cooking before serving to young children, but grated raw carrot and celery may be eaten in salads. Vegetables sold with leaves intact and earth clinging to the roots are more cumbersome, but retain their moisture and freshness longer. Trimmed vegetables will not last so long.

All roots and tubers (e.g. potatoes) should feel smooth and very firm, never flabby, and should be free from blemishes. Old carrots and parsnips are best avoided as the cores of these can be woody. The base of a cabbage, cauliflower, etc., should always be examined. If it looks stained, it is stale; if it is slimy, it is rotten. Peas and beans should be a healthy green, crisp, and not stringy. It is best to choose pods in which the contents are not bulging. Bean sprouts must be absolutely fresh. Fruit-like vegetables, e.g. tomatoes, should be firm, plump and glossy. Any that show the slightest sign of wrinkles, bruising or soft patches should be rejected. The tastiest sweetcorn cobs are densely packed and a pale creamy-yellow; if deep golden, they are over-mature and will taste starchy.

Fruit can generally be divided into four categories; top fruit, soft fruit, citrus fruit and exotic fruit. Top fruit, the term used by fruit growers for all tree fruits, include apples, pears, plums, peaches, cherries, nectarines and nuts. Apples are probably the fruit most popular with children. They should have smooth, unmarked skins. Pears bruise easily and should be handled with care; they are best bought before fully ripe, and ripened at home. Ripe pears will yield when gently pressed at the stalk end. Peaches which have split, or those with bruised skins and brown or soft spots, should be avoided. Cherries should be firm and dry.

Home-grown nuts have the most flavour. It should be remembered, however, that children under the age of two or three years should never be given whole nuts as they occasionally inhale them.

Soft fruits include strawberries, raspberries and currants. They are best used on the day of purchase. All soft fruit, with the exception of gooseberries, leave stains on the bottom of the container. Badly stained containers should be avoided as the fruits are bound to be mushy and often mouldy. The berries should be tipped carefully on to a plate as soon as possible after buying. Any mouldy ones should be picked out and thrown away and the remainder separated on to a tray.

Citrus fruits include grapefruit, lemons and oranges. As all citrus fruit have fairly thick skins, it is sometimes difficult to tell the condition of the fruit. In general, all fruit should have bright, taut and slightly moist skins with a definite aroma. Any that are dry looking or have soft indentations and blemishes on the skin should be avoided.

Exotic fruits include bananas, grapes, pineapples and melons as well as dates, almonds and coconuts. Bananas should be golden yellow, flecked with brown and chosen from a bunch rather than loose. Any with black spots or patches, and damaged or squashy fruits, are best rejected. Grapes should be bought in bunches, if possible. Shrivelled or split berries, or those which show mould near the stems should not be purchased. Ripe melons yield to pressure applied gently at the non-stalk end. Pineapples which are yellowy-green with stiff leaves are ripe. Those which are completely yellow are usually over-ripe.

### Eggs

Up to 95 per cent of eggs come from battery hens, including those labelled 'fresh farm eggs'. Battery hens are frequently kept five to a cage half a metre wide. They lead a monotonous lifestyle, standing for long periods with no natural light. When they want to move, they have to scramble over each other. They can never stretch their wings, fly, perch, walk, scratch the ground or build nests. Battery hens eat inferior food and are encouraged to lay an unnatural number of eggs. Their bones are brittle and fracture easily, and their eggs have shells which are thinner than free-range ones. Free-range hens scratch about and run free, whereas hens that live in deep-litter units, while having more freedom than battery hens, are still confined.

Battery eggs are less nutritious than either free-range or deep-litter eggs. A government investigation into the nutritional composition of different types of eggs found that free-range and deep-litter eggs contain nearly twice as much vitamin $B_{12}$ and slightly more folic acid on average than battery eggs. They also contain more calcium and iron. Free-range eggs are obtainable from farms, health food shops, delicatessens and some large supermarkets. Shops selling genuine free-range eggs are issued with a yellow triangle.

Freshness is important whether buying free-range, deep-litter or battery eggs. The freshest eggs come direct from a producer, the next freshest from large supermarkets, health food shops or the milkman – look out for the date stamp on the box – and the least fresh are generally those from small stores. A fresh egg has a rounded plump yolk, surrounded by a transparent, gelatinous white, with an outer layer of thinner white. The staler the egg, the flatter the yolk and the more the two layers of white mingle and spread in a watery way. Very stale eggs float in water, whereas fresh eggs sink.

## Dairy produce

Most families buy their milk from the milkman. The quality of milk is standardized in degrees of richness. Skimmed milk (blue top) has had virtually all the fat removed – and also the fat-soluble A, D and E vitamins. Semi-skimmed milk is less than 2 per cent fat. Silver top contains an average of 3.8 per cent fat and gold top has a minimum of 4.8 per cent fat. Homogenized milk (red top) has the fat distributed evenly through the milk. Sterilized milk (beer bottle top) and UHT cartons are also available, but do not taste like fresh milk; these keep for a long period until opened.

Cream is usually pasteurized; it is described according to how much butter fat it contains. Half cream contains 12 per cent butter fat, single cream 18 per cent, whipping cream 35 per cent, double cream and extra thick cream 48 per cent, and clotted cream 55 per cent.

Most yoghurts are made with skimmed milk, but full fat milk gives a better taste and is more nutritious. 'Greek' yoghurt is boiled and reduced to give an extra high fat content. All yoghurts are 'live' except those specifically labelled pasteurized.

When buying cheese for children, processed cheeses and cheese spreads should be avoided, as they contain more additives than other cheeses. In general, continental cheeses contain less fat than British ones, but they all contain salt. Nitrites are added to the Dutch cheeses Edam and Gouda. French cheeses are not permitted to contain nitrates or nitrites. Cheese that is sweating greasily, has deep cracks or signs of mould should be avoided.

Butter may be bought salted or unsalted. The unsalted variety does not remain fresh as long as salted butter and is a little more expensive, but is more suitable for children owing to its lower sodium content. Butter wrapped in a transparent cover should not be bought as riboflavin is sensitive to light.

## Meat

Lean meats are preferable to those containing a large proportion of fat. Generally, older animals are fattier than young, the breast or belly is fattier than the leg, and pork is fattier than lamb or beef. Most poultry (except goose and duck), game and offal are lean. Minced meat and sausages are very fatty and so are meat products such as hamburgers and pies. Good-quality mince can, however, make a perfectly nourishing meal as long as most of the fat is removed after cooking. It is worth remembering that the cost of a particular cut of meat is not a reflection of its nutritional value. Beef and veal usually contain small amounts of growth-hormone residues. It is probably a wise precaution to serve lamb to young children more often than beef.

Fresh and frozen meat is not permitted to contain colour, anti-oxidants or preservatives – except mince in Scotland, which may contain added sulphur dioxide. Oven-ready frozen poultry, ham, sausages and hamburgers are usually injected with polyphosphates – these enable the products to retain added water. Butter or extracts of fat from older animals are also sometimes injected into the flesh to improve the flavour.

Cured, pickled or smoked meats, such as bacon, ham, some sausages, luncheon meats, tongue and corned beef are best avoided as these often contain the preservative sodium nitrite – a potential carcinogen. Sausages and prepared beefburgers, etc., which usually contain little meat, a large proportion of fat, refined cereals and the preservative sulphur dioxide, are also unsuitable for children.

## Fish

Choosing fish can be tricky, as freshness is vital. Fresh fish can be recognized by its firm flesh, clear, full and shiny eyes, bright red gills and clean smell. Steaks, cutlets and fillets should have firm, closely packed flakes; any with a fibrous or watery appearance are likely to be stale. Fish whose flesh has a blue or green tinge is almost certainly not fresh – on flat fish this is most apparent on the dark side. Fish can be divided, according to their oil content, into white fish and fatty fish.

In nutritive value fatty fish are superior to white, containing more energy, fat-soluble vitamins A, D and E, and iron. Fatty fish include herring, sardines, mackerel, trout and salmon. Fish oils, unlike animal fat, are high in polyunsaturated fatty acids. These are beneficial to health in that they lower blood cholesterol and make the blood less liable to clot.

Shellfish are not suitable for children as they are frequently responsible for food poisoning and allergies, and often contain excessive amounts of harmful trace elements such as arsenic, cadmium and mercury. White fish, popular with children, include cod, haddock, plaice, whiting and lemon sole. Fish may be bought whole or filleted. The fishmonger is always willing to clean and fillet white fish and remove the head. Fish should always be purchased on the day it is to be eaten.

Freezing fish causes little loss in nutritive value, although some B vitamins and flavours are lost in the drip on thawing. This can be avoided by cooking small pieces of fish without thawing beforehand. It is convenient to buy unbreaded frozen fish portions (available from supermarkets) provided one has the use of a freezer. They may be cooked from frozen without preparation, there is no waste and they are invariably fresher than 'fresh' fish from a fishmonger, which may have been previously frozen.

Smoked and cured fish (smoked haddock, kippers, etc.) are not suitable for children. They are very salty and contain many potentially harmful additives, such as the yellow colouring in smoked haddock and brown (154) in kippers and smoked mackerel, which has been shown to cause genetic mutations in bacteria. Fish-fingers, fishcakes, fish spreads, etc., also contain additives. Furthermore, the breadcrumbs on breaded fish are made from refined flour.

## STORING FRESH FOOD

Many fresh foods if stored correctly remain wholesome for a few days, so shopping need not necessarily be done daily. Vegetables should be stored in the less cold parts of the refrigerator, taking care not to pack them too tightly. Vegetables which have been blanched as they grow (e.g. chicory and leeks) must be protected from light, as must bulbs, roots and tubers. Most fruit, except bananas, keeps best if refrigerated until required. Fruit which needs to be ripened rapidly should be kept at room temperature.

Eggs stay fresh longer if kept in the refrigerator in a covered container. They should be placed with the pointed end downwards, so that the yolk rises towards the air pocket in the rounded end and sustains less damage. Milk, cream, butter and yoghurt should also be stored in the refrigerator.

If butter is to remain outside the refrigerator it must be protected from light to avoid destruction of light-sensitive vitamins. Cheese needs protection from loss of moisture and extreme heat or cold. It should be tightly wrapped (cling film is best), taking care not to trap air in the package, and stored in a cool place. Mouldy cheese should be thrown away.

All meat and fish needs to be stored under refrigeration. Fresh fish should be eaten on the day of purchase or the next day, as it is generally a few days old when bought and goes off much more quickly than meat.

## FOOD LABELLING

Shopping for groceries suitable for inclusion in a child's wholefood diet is difficult if the legislation governing food labelling is not understood.

All pre-packed foods must show the name of the food on the label. Trade marks, brand names or other invented names cannot be used on their own, but only in addition to the proper name of the food. The condition that the food is in must also be stated (e.g. powdered, smoked, dried), and whether it has been treated in any way (e.g. previously frozen). The labelling on most pre-packed foods must include a complete list of ingredients. This shows in descending order of weight the components of the food. Added water need not be included if it does not exceed 5 per cent of the weight of the finished product.

Food manufacturers try to get around this requirement by using several substances with similar biochemical activity in one product. Sugar, for example, which might, if used on its own, constitute the most important ingredient by weight, is often partially replaced by malt, molasses, glucose, honey, etc., which individually come low down on the list of ingredients. At present, the labelling does not have to provide any nutritional information. Foods in very small packages need not have a list of ingredients.

Food additives are usually listed by category names – e.g. colours, emulsifiers – which explain what they are used for. In many cases this name will be followed by the additive's chemical name or serial number or both. For example: 'flavour enhancer – monosodium glutamate' or 'preservative – E200'. Serial numbers which begin with the letter E are given to those additives which are generally recognized by the EEC as safe. Certain other additives used in the UK have a serial number without the prefix 'E' as they have not yet been generally approved.

Most foods are date-marked. The main exceptions are long-life foods. Usually the date mark is in the form of 'best before' followed by the day, month and year. The year may be omitted if the food will not remain at its best for longer than three months. The day may be omitted if the food will remain at its best for more than three months; the phrase used then is 'best before end', followed by the month and year. Perishable foods, like yoghurt, which are intended to be eaten within six weeks of packing, may alternatively be marked with the words 'Sell by', followed by the latest recommended date of sale, expressed in terms of a day and month. The label should also indicate that the food is best eaten within a certain number of days of purchase.

## SHOPPING FOR HEALTH FOODS

Since food is one of the main expenses in the household budget, parents are understandably concerned about how much it is going to cost. Health-food shops sell organically grown vegetables – often at higher prices than one would pay for conventionally grown vegetables obtained from greengrocers – and charge high prices for vitamin pills and other dietary supplements. This has led to a common belief that wholefoods cost more than the standard British diet. In fact a well-balanced wholefood diet is often cheaper than the standard diet, since one can eliminate or restrict many expensive refined foods. Furthermore, time and money is saved in terms of less frequent visits to doctors and dentists, and fewer prescriptions.

Buying food from health-food shops does not automatically guarantee that the food is suitable for inclusion in a child's diet. The wholefood shopper is sometimes led astray by the growing array of 'health-food junk', so labels must always be read, even if mother nature herself is depicted on the package. Statements such as 'enriched' and 'fortified' should be regarded with suspicion. The best guideline for buying wholefoods is to select those foods which are as close as possible to their natural state e.g. brown rice, fresh fruit and vegetables, pulses, nuts, etc. This means avoiding those foods whose integrity has been disturbed, e.g. white flour, canned fruit, ready-prepared meals.

Although almost all supermarkets and some grocers now sell some wholefoods, e.g. dried pulses, dried fruit, etc., the widest range of products is still obtainable from specialist shops. Products available from health-food shops include whole grains, 100 per cent stone-ground, organic wholemeal bread, gluten-free bread, wholegrain pastas, dried fruit, seeds, unsalted nuts, free-range eggs, sugar-free jams and marmalades, unhydrogenated nut butters, low-salt yeast extracts, concentrated sugar-free apple juice, healthier snack products, soya products, dried sea vegetables and organically grown vegetables and fruit, as well as vitamins, cosmetics, etc.

Parents can begin to take advantage of the range of health foods currently available as soon as the baby begins to eat solid food.

A baby's first cereal is usually rice, as this is considered to be the least allergenic of the grains. Commercial 'baby' rice is made from refined white rice and is depleted of fibre and many vitamins and should be avoided. Wholegrain ground rice, rice flour or rice flakes are a far superior food and are available at most health-food shops. Salt-free, sugar-free brown puffed rice cakes are a healthy alternative to commercial 'rusks' and are very popular with young babies. All cereals may be eaten by babies older than six months. These include wheat, rye, barley, oats, maize, buckwheat and millet, as well as rice. Flour or flakes made from these grains are very easy to cook and need no further preparation. Koh-koh is a nutritious unrefined baby cereal made from whole grains and pulses. Some health-food shops stock it.

Whole grains can be bought in bulk for convenience and cheapness. They will keep indefinitely in dry, rodent-proof conditions. Wholegrain flours should be purchased in small quantities as they tend to go rancid, rot very quickly and are liable to infestation. That is to say that, unlike refined flours, they support life.

Bread made from organically grown wheat is best for young

children. It is relatively free from chemical fertilizers, pesticide residues and food additives. Ordinary wholemeal bread may contain higher levels of pesticide than white bread since the chemicals accumulate in the bran layers. This is an example of the extra care that must be taken when eating a wholefood diet. Where a choice is available between organically grown grains and non-organic grains, it is worth choosing the organic varieties in spite of the extra expense.

Wholewheat pastas such as lasagne, macaroni and spaghetti make a nourishing and satisfying alternative to white pasta. The packet must specify 100 per cent wholewheat. Sugar-free tomato ketchup is also available.

Health-food shops stock a wide range of dried fruit. Some are treated with the preservative sulphur dioxide (E220). Although the quantity is seldom great enough to be toxic, it is present in amounts well within the allergy-causing range in susceptible children. Dried fruits which usually contain sulphur dioxide include apple rings, apricots, peaches and pears. Unsulphured fruit is available and this must be declared. Raisins may be coated with mineral oil (a carcinogen) unless it is stated that they contain vegetable oil, or are oil-free. Banana chips and pineapple pieces are sometimes coated with sugar or honey and these should be avoided. All dried fruit should be rinsed in hot water and dried before consumption.

Unsalted, shelled nuts, such as almonds, brazils, cashews, coconut, hazelnuts, peanuts and walnuts are indispensable for wholefood and vegetarian cooking. Whole nuts must not be given to children under three years, however, as there is a risk that they may inhale them and choke. Crushed nuts or nut powders are suitable for younger children. Pumpkin and sunflower seeds are popular with children, so are 'mixes' such as mixed fruit, mixed fruit and nuts, and 'trail mix'. Seeds have been known to cause intestinal obstruction when very large quantities are eaten, so these should be limited.

Most dried beans and lentils (pulses) are suitable in small quantities for children over one year if prepared properly. Even babies under one year may eat them if they are well cooked, blended and sieved to remove husks. Aduki, black-eye and butter beans, chick peas, flageolet beans, lentils, mung, pinto, red kidney and soya beans and split peas are just some of the pulse varieties available. Some children, however, suffer digestive problems if certain varieties are eaten, especially the longer cooking ones, e.g. soya beans. All pulses, but particularly red kidney beans, must be boiled for ten minutes at the beginning of the cooking period, in order to destroy harmful substances present in the pulses.

Choosing a breakfast cereal can be confusing, as many so-called 'healthy' cereals contain sugar, albeit in the form of raw sugar or honey. All-Bran, for example, has 21 per cent of its calories in the form of sugars, and many cereals contain more salt than potato crisps. Of the major commercial cereals, only Shredded Wheat, Cubs and Puffed Wheat are prepared from the whole grain and do not contain salt or sugar.

Muesli is a good nutritious breakfast cereal and can be finely ground using a food processor or liquidizer and then left to soak overnight to make it more digestible for younger children. Packeted muesli contains dried fruit, chopped or flaked nuts and one or two cereal grains (usually oats). The ingredients should be checked and an unsweetened brand selected. If none can be found then it is best made at home. Once children acquire a taste for sweetened muesli they are loath to change to the unsweetened varieties. Fresh fruit may be added to breakfast cereals but never sugar or honey.

Natural fruit jams are a boon to a wholefood diet. Standard jams are about two thirds sugar by weight, whereas natural fruit jams are one third natural fruit sugars. Apple juice is usually used as a sweetener. Apple-juice-sweetened jams contain no artificial colours, flavours or preservatives and are available in the following flavours: strawberry, raspberry, cherry, apricot, blackcurrant, hedgerow fruits, mixed berry and orange marmalade.

Apple and pear spread is made purely from apples and pears and contains no other ingredients. It cannot be considered to be a wholefood however, as the fruit has been stripped of most of its fibre and, owing to its concentration, it may contribute significantly to the sugar content of the diet. Honey may be 'natural' but it contains about 75 per cent sugar and the rest is almost all water. Alternatives to spread on a child's bread are natural peanut butter and other nut spreads, sunflower spread and sesame spread; they are not only sugar-free and often salt-free but are extremely nutritious when combined with wholemeal bread. Most commercial peanut butters (found in supermarkets) have been partly artificially saturated (hydrogenated) and contain sugar, salt and additives.

In general, yeast extracts (e.g. Marmite) are not suitable for children due to their extremely high salt content. There is now available, however, a 'low-salt' yeast extract (Natex) which contains less than 10 per cent the amount of salt present in other similar-tasting extracts.

Biscuits and cakes are not 'good' for a child just because they come from a health-food shop and they should only be allowed occasionally. Raw sugar or brown sugar is just as harmful as white sugar, so when selecting these foods it is particularly important to read the labels carefully. If sugar, honey, etc., is first or second in the list of ingredients they should not be purchased. Furthermore, many which claim to be 'sugar free' – sugar referring to sucrose only – list molasses, honey, malt, dextrose or syrup as ingredients. 'Wholefood' biscuits are, however, infinitely preferable to most supermarket cakes and biscuits since they are generally made from the whole grain, are free from additives such as colouring and chemical preservatives, and often contain highly nutritious ingredients such as nuts and seeds, and carob instead of chocolate.

Savoury snacks, so popular with children, are best bought in health-food shops, as they stock additive-free wholegrain snacks. These snacks should, however, only rarely be permitted as they always contain salt.

Sea vegetables, which can be found in health-food shops, are rich in minerals, especially iodine. Many different types of sea vegetable are now available; the best known of these is kelp. Kelp powder can be used to flavour soups, stews and casseroles. Carragheen moss is a sea vegetable with amazing gelling power that can be used instead of gelatine. Agar is a powdered form of seaweed gelling agent. *Nori* are paper-thin sheets of dried seaweed. *Kombu* can be cooked in water for a few minutes to make a good stock. *Arame* are fine shreds of seaweed which can be cooked as a vegetable, or added like noodles to soups. *Wakame* is used like *arame* and can also be used to make laver bread, the traditional Welsh dish. All cured seaweeds must be avoided as these contain nitrite.

Many health-food shops are outlets for organically grown vegetables. Organic produce is grown without the use of synthetically produced chemicals – artificial fertilizers or pesticides. Organic farming improves the structure of the soil and is less harmful to the environment than current conventional methods. Organic foods are more expensive, yields are usually reduced and more of the crop is lost to pests; soil fertility is, however, maintained. Non-organic food costs less, but depletes the wealth of the land and is potentially hazardous to health.

The disadvantage of eating organic foods is that the growth of moulds is more common on these foods than on those that have been treated with fungicides. The poisons produced by some moulds may rarely induce cancer. Furthermore, organic food is not always pollutant-free: radioactive fallout, and chemicals from tractor exhausts, can be deposited equally on both organic and ordinary food, and pesticides and chemicals which have entered the water supply can contaminate crops.

# 8

# BREAST- OR BOTTLE-FEEDING

Until the early years of this century, there was no choice in how to feed the new-born baby. If, for any reason, the mother could not or did not want to breast-feed, a wetnurse had to be found. Infant foods based on cows' milk have only been available in this country this century, and before the Second World War their use was comparatively rare. Although the number of artificial baby milks (infant formulas) on the market has increased, as has the number of bottle-fed babies, breast-feeding is now regaining popularity.

Baby-milk manufacturers encourage mothers to bottle-feed by providing free samples of milk in hospitals and baby clinics. Mothers then get the impression that the health authorities endorse bottle-feeding, and they may either never start to breast-feed their babies, or switch to bottle-feeding once they get home from hospital.

## BREAST-FEEDING

It used to be thought that the advantages of breast milk were few. It was not surprising then, that when artificial foods derived from cows' milk were first produced, both mothers and the medical profession thought that these were as good if not better than breast milk.

All mammals suckle their young and the composition of the milk they produce is as variable as the diets they consume. During the long period of evolution, the mother's milk has adapted to the needs of the young and the type of milk produced takes into account the animal's growth rate, type of digestive tract, its natural illnesses and so on.

Recent research has emphasized that, in composition, human milk is a much more suitable food for babies than even the most carefully modified preparations of cows' milk. If an infant is born well-nourished and has adequate exposure to sunlight – providing vitamin D which is lacking in breast milk – human milk from a healthy mother in sufficient quantity will supply all his nutritional needs for optimal growth and health for the first six months after birth. Human milk, but not infant formula, has a built-in protection against infection and varies in composition throughout the feed. Breast-feeding is also thought to protect against many diseases in later life, and this is hardly surprising when one considers that over time mother's milk has adapted to the needs of the baby.

### Some good reasons for breast-feeding

The benefits of breast-feeding are seemingly endless, but perhaps the most important is the protection it gives against disease. First colostrum (early milk), and then milk, protects a baby from infection by viruses, bacteria, yeasts and other organisms. Gastroenteritis (infective diarrhoea) for example, a potentially fatal disease, is relatively rare amongst totally breast-fed babies, but is frequently seen in bottle-feeders, and often leads to hospitalization. Common respiratory infections – colds, ear infections, coughs, flu and pneumonia – are also less frequent, as are tetanus, measles, mumps, polio, meningitis and many other diseases.

Exposure to 'foreign' proteins at a time when the body's immunological mechanisms are likely to be immature may be a significant factor in the development of chronic allergic illness which can continue into later life. The first 'foreign' protein to which infants are usually exposed is cows' milk, although it may be any food. To reduce the incidence of allergic disease, particularly in babies of allergic parents, the mother should fully breast-feed her baby for four months. Sensitization to foods which may cause allergy (allergens) may also occur, however, in fully breast-fed infants; presumably the allergen is secreted in the breast milk.

Allergy to cows' milk may cause eczema, diarrhoea, vomiting, failure to thrive, colic, asthma, nettle rash, runny nose, cough and wheezing. Sometimes babies are given a surreptitious bottle feed in the hospital nursery by nursing staff during the first hours after birth. This practice is well meant, but ill advised and it may entirely nullify the benefits – as regards protection against allergies – of subsequent exclusive breast-feeding.

Breast-fed babies almost never become overweight – a major

health hazard. Furthermore, fat babies have a significantly greater chance of being fat in childhood, adolescence or adult life than do thin babies. Cot deaths are less common amongst babies who are being breast-fed and constipation is unknown. The breast-fed baby is less likely to suffer from dental decay when he is older and will have a better jaw and mouth development and straighter teeth than a bottle-feeder. This is because breast-feeders do not have the abnormal swallowing mechanism that a bottle-fed baby learns when sucking from the bottle teat.

A breast-fed baby's stools have a less strong smell than those produced by bottle-fed babies, and he is less likely to suffer from nappy rash. Furthermore, if a breast-fed baby regurgitates any milk, there is no unpleasant smell, whereas a bottle-fed baby's vomit has a foul, sour smell which can quickly permeate the clothing of both the baby and mother. Breast-feeding helps the mother to get her figure back to normal more quickly. It saves time, costs nothing – except for the small amount of extra food a breast-feeding mother needs – and breast milk is always available at the right temperature, so the baby need not be kept waiting.

There are many other benefits of breast-feeding, too numerous to mention, but it is obvious why exclusive breast-feeding is the 'ideal' start in life for a baby and most convenient for the mother. The only serious disadvantage of breast-feeding in this country is probably the frustration and hunger suffered by a baby whose mother has inadequate milk for him. This is almost always easily overcome, however, with help and perseverance. (See also The Working Mother, p. 139.)

### How to breast-feed successfully

As long as the baby is healthy and there is no medical reason why a woman should not breast-feed, she can almost always make a success of it providing there is sufficient motivation. All mammals provide their young with a complete food which is unique to the species. Man is no exception. First colostrum, then transitional milk and later mature milk can completely satisfy all the infant's needs during the early months after birth.

Human milk may, however, contain a number of substances derived from maternal blood which have no nutritive or protective value for the infant. These include some hormones, drugs, pollutants or contaminants. In general, the risk of any harm is outweighed by the benefits of breast-feeding. Nevertheless it is advisable to avoid excessive consumption of certain foods while breast-feeding, such as cows' milk, which may cause allergy in the baby, and beverages such as coffee and alcohol; and to smoke only in moderation, if at all. Caffeine, nicotine and alcohol have all been shown to pass into milk and may affect the baby. Alcohol and nicotine may reduce the milk supply and may oblige the mother to abandon breast-feeding through lack of milk. Nearly all medicines, including the contraceptive pill, pass into breast milk and medical advice should be sought before taking any drugs.

The early days are very important if breast-feeding is to be successful, particularly if the birth took place in hospital. Getting the baby latched on to the areola which surrounds the nipple is the primary concern and it is vital that help is obtained until this is achieved. Ideally, the baby should remain with the mother, but if he is taken away to the nursery, she must insist that he is brought in for feeding as soon as he cries and must not be given anything at all to drink, even if it is only water or sugar water. Babies breast-fed on demand do not need extra water or any other fluid unless ordered for medical reasons. Sugar water may harm the pancreas by stimulating the outflow of insulin too early in life, or even cause allergies later on.

Colostrum (for the first few days) and then milk satisfies the nutritional needs of the very young infant as well as providing invaluable protection against infection. Complementing the feed with infant formula during the early days will undermine the mother's confidence and cause her to produce less milk than she would have done had the baby been allowed to suckle freely. Furthermore, it is so easy for the baby to drink from a teat, that he may not want to return to the breast when he finds he has to work harder to get his milk from it.

A baby should be fed 'on demand' rather than at fixed feeding times. This allows frequent stimulation of the breast and nipple, ensuring the continued secretion of prolactin for milk production and oxytocin for the milk ejection or 'let-down' reflex. It should be emphasized to first-time mothers that during the early days of breast-feeding, the number of feeds required 'on demand' may be as many as ten to twelve, or even more, in twenty-four hours, although this number will be reduced as breast-feeding becomes established.

Feeding a newborn baby at fixed four-hourly intervals is unlikely to lead to the establishment of successful breast-feeding. Inadequate breast-feeding usually results in a discontented crying baby, but he may remain quiet and, if allowed, may sleep for long intervals between feeds and during the night. Weight gain will be unsatisfactory. In such cases, the baby must be woken for his feeds if he is to thrive. Long gaps between feeds may also result in a baby with colic. This is because he is often so hungry by the time he is fed that he swallows air with his milk and it causes pain as it passes through his intestines.

Mothers sometimes give up breast-feeding after only a token effort because of physical problems. Sore nipples are a very common complaint. This can usually be prevented or cured by rubbing a small amount of vitamin E oil into the nipples after a feed. The less sore nipple should always be offered first and the breasts left exposed to the air after every feed. Painful engorgement can be relieved by expressing milk or by feeding the baby more often.

Getting the baby to take the breast can sometimes cause problems because of inverted or poorly protractile nipples. Maternity wards will, if requested, provide a mechanical aid to attach to the breast through which the baby can suck. This may be used at the beginning of the feed, until the nipple protrudes enough for the baby to get hold of. Eventually, with feeding, the nipples will begin to protrude more, and these aids may be discarded. If all else fails, then it is better to express milk with a breast pump and feed the baby with breast milk from a bottle than to resort to infant formula. Sick or handicapped babies who are unable to suck from the breast may also be successfully breast-fed in this way.

Sometimes breast-feeding is successful in hospital but fails when the mother gets home. In these circumstances help may be sought from the community midwife, health visitor or the local branch of the National Childbirth Trust or the La Leche League.

Many mothers give up breast-feeding because of insufficient milk and a few of these stop in the first three days, even though they could not be expected to produce milk so soon. It is important to remember that the more often the baby is put to the breast, the more milk will be produced. Provided that the baby looks healthy, is putting on weight and seems content, and the mother is eating a nourishing diet and has given up smoking and heavy drinking, he is probably getting enough to eat.

Breast milk is lacking in vitamin D and to prevent the possible development of rickets, a breast-fed baby should be given a daily vitamin D supplement (e.g. Children's Vitamin Drops) starting when he is one month old.

A baby should be fully breast-fed for at least four months, and partially breast-fed until six months, when he can begin to drink diluted cows' milk. When he is about four months old solid food and water from a cup may be given. By following this regime, bottles need never be used, and the problem of weaning the baby off the breast and then off the bottle is avoided.

## Changing from breast-feeding to bottle-feeding

Some mothers start by breast-feeding their babies, but give it up long before a baby can obtain all his fluid from a cup (six to nine months). The switch from breast-feeding to bottle-feeding should take place over a couple of weeks so that the baby has time to adjust and the breast milk has a chance to dry up. Engorgement can occur even in women who are giving up breast-feeding because of insufficient milk.

To give up breast-feeding, a bottle of infant formula should be substituted for the feed at which the mother has least milk. After a few days, or when the breasts are comfortable, another breast-feed should be dropped and so on until eventually all the feeds are given from a bottle. Some mothers choose to breast-feed partially, at night for example, to save having to heat up the bottle. This can be successful provided milk is still being produced.

## Expressing breast milk

When a baby feeds at the breast, he draws the nipple into his mouth and suckles on the dark coloured skin, the areola, surrounding the nipple. After a few seconds the mother can tell that the baby is getting milk. But the breast can also be encouraged to give up milk without a baby actually suckling. This is known as expressing breast milk.

Learning to express breast milk can be vital right from the start. If the baby is premature, for example, he may be tube-fed in hospital with breast milk. It is also very useful if the mother's breasts become engorged and she wants to relieve the painful pressure between or just before feeds. Sometimes the baby may be sleepy or not very well and does not want to feed for long. The breast-milk supply can then be maintained by emptying the breasts after he has finished his feed.

If the mother is separated from her baby for a short time because of illness or some other crisis, she can continue to produce breast milk by expressing it as many times each day as she was breast-feeding. Some mothers choose to be away from their baby for one or more of the breast-feeds in the day. Milk can be expressed either after a feed or between feeds and then stored until used. A working mother can express milk at work and then leave breast milk for the child-minder to give her baby during the day.

Milk can be expressed by hand, by gently massaging the breast towards the nipple, but this is very time-consuming and tiring. Various mechanical methods have been designed to overcome this problem. The breast is stimulated into delivering milk by creating a partial vacuum around the nipple – a gentle sucking. The three types of pump which do this are the bulb hand pump, the syringe hand pump and the electric pump. Care should be taken not to damage the nipple by over-enthusiastic expressing.

Cleanliness is of the utmost importance when expressing milk to feed a baby. Equipment should be prepared for use by washing well, rubbing the feeding teats with salt, sterilizing and then rinsing with boiled water. If the mother prefers not to give her baby a bottle, he can be fed by cup and spoon for all those feeds he does not get directly from suckling at the breast.

Breast milk must be stored properly. If left out of the refrigerator it will rapidly breed germs, and could make the baby ill. Milk should be expressed into a sterilized bottle and the top sealed. It is unwise to keep milk much longer than forty-eight hours under refrigeration. Milk can be frozen for up to six months, but a sterile, sealed plastic container should be used and the milk consumed immediately after thawing.

## BOTTLE-FEEDING

Only a very small number of women are genuinely unable to breast-feed, but some babies cannot digest or tolerate human milk due to prematurity, abnormal physiological conditions, etc., and alternatives are required. The majority of women who bottle-feed their babies, however, do so for personal reasons.

Cows' milk, and preparations made from it, are the usual sub-stitute for human milk. Cows' milk was chosen as the breast-milk substitute not because it is the nearest in composition to human milk – donkey milk is much closer – but because of the existence in the Western world of herds of cows which are already being reared for meat and dairy produce. Provided the parents are educated in home hygiene and the family is able to afford the cost of these preparations, a baby can be successfully reared on these artificial foods.

Cows' milk cannot be given to very young infants (under six months of age) unless it has been processed. Compared with human milk, it contains more protein, more minerals, less lactose and about the same quantity of fat. Many commercial cows'-milk-based products are available. Such artificial feeds, known as infant formulas, are usually sold in powder form. In all of them the content of protein and sodium is much less than in natural cows' milk and approaches that in human milk; the calcium and phosphorus content is also reduced. All have added sugar, usually lactose (milk sugar), but often other sugars which are much sweeter than lactose and encourage babies to develop a sweet tooth at an early age. In some, the butter fat has been replaced by vegetable oils and animal fats. All are fortified with vitamin D to much higher concentrations than those found in either cows' milk or human milk.

No technological advance, however, has produced a cows'-milk-based product as suitable for a baby as breast milk. The long-term effects on a baby's health from this relatively 'new' artificial food are not yet known. Many mothers appear to be under the misapprehension that although breast milk is better for babies than infant formula, these formulas do not actually do any harm.

A bottle-fed baby is less likely to achieve optimum health, either during infancy or in later life, and his growth rate may not be ideal. The introduction of infant formulas has undoubtedly contributed to the rise in Western diseases, but until medical research conclusively quantifies the health risks associated with these foods, mothers will continue to feed their babies these inferior products.

Dried milk powders are convenient, since a mother can buy two or three weeks' supply, which can easily be stored. As bacteria cannot grow on dry powders, these are much safer than liquid preparations. The most important products of the dairy industry which are used in the manufacture of infant formulas are cows' milk; skimmed milk – a byproduct of butter manufacture which contains all the nutrients of cows' milk except fat and fat-soluble vitamins; whey – a byproduct of cheese manufacture; and demineralized whey – whey

from which most of the minerals have been removed. Other substances which are used in the manufacture of some infant formulas
are not products of the dairy industry. These include maltodextrins
(sweetening agents), vegetable oils, animal fats, mineral salts and
vitamins.

There are two main types of complete infant formulas based on
cows' milk. The first type are skimmed milk formulas with added
carbohydrate and fats, examples of which are:

Cow & Gate Plus (added lactose)
Milumil (added maltodextrin and
  starch)
SMA (added lactose)

In these infant formulas the protein is unmodified cows' milk
protein, the fat is a mixture of vegetable oils and animal fats, and the
carbohydrate is lactose from the skimmed milk to which is added
either more lactose, or maltodextrin and starch. The concentration
of protein and minerals is reduced compared with cows' milk. The
fat composition resembles that of human milk fat more closely than
does the fat in cows' milk.

The second type of infant formula is more expensive and consists
of skimmed milk with demineralized whey and mixed fats;
examples are:

Aptamil
Cow & Gate Premium
SMA Gold Cap

A small amount of skimmed milk is used with demineralized whey,
to which a mixture of vegetable oils and animal fats is added. The
cows' milk protein has been modified so that it is more like human
milk. The fat composition resembles human milk fat more closely
than does the fat in cows' milk. The carbohydrate is lactose from
skimmed milk and demineralized whey. The use of demineralized
whey in these formulas permits the mineral content to be reduced
and to approach the average concentrations found in mature human
milk. All the above-mentioned formulas may be used as 'complete'
feeds.

These 'humanized' formulas have a lower sodium content than
the less modified feeds, and while there is little doubt that low
mineral feeds may be of value in reducing the incidence of salt
poisoning in infancy, the same ends may be achieved by accurately

reconstituting feeds, avoiding the use of solids in the first three to four months, and satisfying thirst with water, not milk.

The main disadvantage of these feeds appears to be that de-mineralization – the process by which the mineral content of cows' milk is reduced – may decrease the amounts of certain trace elements present in the milk. Although these can be restored, in-adequate knowledge of the infant's requirements of trace elements, and of their availability in various chemical forms, means that any restoration may be incomplete.

There is no firm evidence to suggest that formulas containing demineralized whey are nutritionally superior to other milk-based formulas for the normal infant. They do, however, appear to be of a high nutritional quality and are likely to be preferable in certain instances. A mother should ask the maternity hospital, clinic or her GP if a demineralized formula is necessary for her baby. Whichever formula a baby is fed he should be given it (in addition to solids after four months) until he is at least six months old, when household milk is suitable.

Follow-on formulas, which are manufactured for babies of four to six months and older who have started solid feeding, do not meet DHSS requirements for milks for babies under six months and should be avoided.

Some infants are intolerant of cows' milk and they are usually fed on an adequate soya-based milk substitute. Before switching from a cows' milk formula to a soya-based one, however, a doctor's advice must be sought. Soya-based formulas are not as good nutritionally as cows' milk formulas, and their indiscriminate use for vague symptoms and signs not proved to be due to cows' milk intolerance is to be avoided. Furthermore, the allegation that soya milks are less allergenic than cows' milk has not been confirmed, and soya-based formula feeding is said to result in poor antibody responses to immunization with polio virus, diphtheria, pertussis and tetanus vaccines. Examples of some soya-based milk substitutes that are suitable as the sole source of nourishment of young infants are:

| | |
|---|---|
| Formula S Soya Food | Wysoy |
| Pro Sobee | |

These are free of lactose as well as milk protein. Since they are entirely of plant origin, they are acceptable to vegetarians and vegans. These infant formulas must be differentiated, however, from some other soya-based milk preparations (available in health-food shops), which may not meet the requirements of either young infants, or older infants and pre-school children.

Goats' milk (and ewes' milk) are not recommended for infants under six months of age. Modified goats' milk could be used under extreme circumstances, for example in cows'-milk-protein intolerance, when all other alternatives have been exhausted. Medical advice should be sought on how to modify goats' milk.

### Giving feeds

When dried infant formulas are correctly mixed and used according to the manufacturer's instructions, they will adequately satisfy a baby's needs. Hospitals use ready-prepared feeds for convenience. These are more expensive than powdered milks and are not available to the public. The same brand of milk, made up from powder, sometimes looks and smells slightly different from the prepared bottles available in hospitals. The milk, however, contains exactly the same constituents, and the apparent differences are only due to the way the milk is made up.

The feed must always be made up precisely according to instructions, with the scoop provided with the particular brand of milk. If the mixture is made stronger than the directions indicate, the milk will be over-concentrated and may cause the baby to become dehydrated if no extra water is given. This is because in infancy the kidneys are less efficient than in adulthood, requiring more water to eliminate excess sodium, potassium and urea (the waste products of unwanted protein in the diet). Dehydration often causes the baby to cry and the mother may respond by giving more feed, rather than water, so increasing the accumulation of waste products. Convulsions and brain damage may follow. Diarrhoea, which causes severe loss of water from the body, also exacerbates dehydration.

Over-concentrating a feed may result in obesity, as will the addition of cereals or sugar to the bottle. If the feed is made up weaker than directed, the baby will not get enough nourishment.

When making up a feed the following rules should be observed: hands must be washed before making up bottles; the correct number of scoops must be used as directed on the packet; the scoops must never be packed but should be levelled off with a clean knife. Bottles, teats and bottle brushes should be thoroughly cleaned every time they are used and bottles and teats sterilized by using one of the special hypochlorite preparations available at the chemist. After each feed, the bottle should be rinsed in cold water, washed with detergent and a bottle brush, and rinsed again thoroughly. The teat should be rinsed in cold soapy water or rinsed and then rubbed inside and outside with salt to remove the milk scum. Bottles, etc., should be left completely immersed in the special solution until they are wanted and then rinsed in boiled water.

Domestic water which has been artificially softened, or water which has been repeatedly boiled, should not be used in the reconstitution of a baby's feeds, since it will have a high sodium (salt) content. Sodium is closely linked with water in the body and an imbalance of either can be serious and even fatal. Water from the hot tap should never be used as this contains higher lead levels than mains water. In areas where nitrate levels are elevated, bottled spring water should be used for reconstituting feeds.

To make up a bottle, the required quantity of warm (previously boiled) water is measured into a sterilized bottle, and the specified number of scoops of powder added. The cap is placed on the bottle and the bottle shaken well until the powder is dissolved. The teat is then put on the bottle and the temperature of the milk checked before feeding by shaking a few drops on to the wrist to ensure that it is only lukewarm. The bottle should be shaken occasionally during the feed.

Alternatively, the total amount of water may be measured into a sterilized jug. Using the scoop provided in the packet, the required number of level scoops of powder is added to the water and stirred well with a sterilized fork. The milk is immediately transferred to sterilized feeding bottles and the capped bottles stored in a refrigerator until required. When needed, each bottle is shaken gently, stood in hot water to warm the food to the correct temperature, then shaken again. Unfinished feeds should never be saved and only enough feeds for one day should be made up. To avoid the incubation of bacteria in what is effectively an excellent culture medium, vacuum flasks and insulators should not be used to keep feeds warm for more than a few minutes before feeding.

In the early days, the baby should be offered milk whenever he seems to be hungry, and the feeding stopped when eager sucking ceases. A schedule will gradually evolve out of the baby's digestive pattern, given that it takes three to four hours for a baby to digest a full feed. If the baby appears to be hungry he should be offered a greater volume of feed, or more feeds per day, not a more concentrated feed.

In the UK, formula feeding is continued until the baby is at least six months, and sometimes a year old. When the baby starts drinking household milk, a vitamin D supplement (Children's Vitamin Drops, or cod-liver oil) should be given.

# 9

# WEANING

Weaning begins when breast- or bottle-feeding is replaced by a mixed diet. It should be a gradual process, which extends over a period of weeks or even months, and there is no hard and fast rule for its commencement.

## WHEN TO START SOLIDS

The age at which solid foods are introduced varies from a few weeks until the end of the baby's first or even second year. In most parts of the world, solids are not introduced until towards the end of the first year, but in Europe and North America their early introduction is fashionable.

A normal, full-term baby's nutritional needs can be entirely met until four to six months of age by milk and sunshine alone. Some babies may thrive on this regimen until they are eight months old. Failure to introduce solids by six months, however, may lead to an inadequate supply of energy and particularly iron. In developing countries, where mixed feeding is introduced late in the first year, or even the second, weight gain is comparable with that of Western infants at three months, but falls dramatically after that. This is due to the inadequacy of milk alone as a suitable diet after the first few months.

Medical opinion suggests that mixed feeding may be initiated between four and six months of age, and starting it any earlier than this adds unnecessary risks. Signs that a baby may be ready to accept solid foods include showing an interest in what people are eating, the eruption of teeth, and the mouthing of objects. If he rejects puréed food, however, then mixed feeding should be delayed a little longer.

## RISKS ASSOCIATED WITH THE EARLY
## INTRODUCTION OF SOLIDS

Despite recommendations that mixed feeding should not be started too early, over 96 per cent of mothers in Britain introduce solids by the time their babies reach four months of age. Some start when the baby is less than a month old. Not only are they substituting a nutritionally inferior product (solids) for a superior one (breast milk or adequate formula), but many nutritional problems arise due to early or excessive use of solids.

Obesity, which sometimes persists into adulthood, is common in babies fed solids too early. Baby foods used in the first four months are mainly highly sweetened cereal preparations, fruit syrups and rusks. Babies like these pleasant foods, and it is easy to understand why a mother may give them in excessive quantities.

Salt poisoning is a hazard when sodium-rich weaning foods are offered too early, or concentrated milk feeds are given. Infant kidneys are not as mature as those of older children and they sometimes cannot excrete this excess salt. Dehydration then follows, and if this condition is allowed to continue, permanent damage to the brain may occur.

Early introduction of solids – before four months – increases the risk of allergic disease, due to the immaturity of the baby's digestive system. Foods particularly likely to cause problems include wheat, egg, cows' milk, and products made from them such as rusks, cheese, butter, yoghurt, etc., and these foods should not be introduced until the baby is six months old.

Wheat and, to a small extent, rye, barley and oats, but not rice, contain the protein gluten, and their consumption in early infancy may cause the onset of coeliac disease – a severe food allergy – in susceptible infants. An infant with coeliac disease fails to thrive, loses his appetite and is apathetic, pale, irritable and pot-bellied. He passes large, pale, offensive, soft stools. Children suffering from coeliac disease must be on a gluten-free diet, usually for life. It is a sensible precaution not to introduce these cereals into the baby's diet until he is six months old. Rice is considered to be the least allergenic cereal and may be introduced at four months.

Allergies to egg are usually caused by raw or undercooked egg whites. The best way to introduce eggs is to hard-boil them, and to offer the baby small amounts of the yolk. If it is well tolerated, hard-boiled white, uncooked yolk, soft-boiled egg and whole scrambled egg can be introduced.

Pasteurized or boiled cows' milk may be given when the baby is six to nine months old. Fresh milk only should be used (the date should be checked on the foil top) and it should be well-diluted at first with cooled boiled water to make it more easily digestible. Sometimes a baby will vomit when first fed cows' milk. This is usually because the milk has not been diluted enough. Mothers should resist the temptation to substitute soya-based milk for cows' milk unless a genuine allergy to cows' milk has been diagnosed. Goats' milk may be given to allergic babies over six months old as a possible alternative to fresh cows' milk. It should be boiled for two minutes (most goats' milk is sold unpasteurized) and then diluted to three-quarter strength.

## HOW TO WEAN A BABY

The introduction of solid foods and the gradual replacement of milk provides nutrients such as iron, which may be lacking in the milk. It is possible to wean a baby on to foods that the rest of the family are eating, and this is the usual practice in most countries. In the Western world, where there is no shortage of food, specially developed weaning foods are largely a convenience, although they sometimes offer a better guarantee of good nutrition if the mother has little or no knowledge of nutritional principles.

During the process of weaning, the baby will make the transition from numerous breast or bottle feeds to three meals a day. Unlimited breast milk or an adequate infant formula are complete foods and provide all the nutrients needed by the young baby. During the early stages of weaning, therefore, there is no need to worry whether the baby is getting a balanced diet as long as he is having breast or bottle feeds. Once solids begin to form a significant part of the diet, or he starts drinking diluted household milk (after six months), more attention will need to be paid to what he is eating.

To start weaning, tiny tastes of puréed foods are offered on a teaspoon, but only after the baby has had a breast or bottle feed. Solid food must not be allowed to crowd out milk at this stage. Between four and six months, suitable foods include most properly prepared meat, white fish, fruit, vegetables and rice. A small amount of fat or a fatty food (in addition to milk) should be included in the diet as soon as the baby is eating more than a few teaspoons of food a day. Fat is rich in the energy a young baby needs and acts as a vehicle for fat-soluble vitamins. Most meats are high in fat. On days when meat is not served, however, half a teaspoon of cold-pressed, polyunsaturated vegetable oil should be given. After six months a wider range of foods may be eaten, including all cereals, pasteurized cows' milk, yoghurt, cheese, butter, eggs, etc.

In order to be able to identify foods which cause adverse reactions, such as diarrhoea, vomiting, colic, asthma, a rash, etc., it is a sensible precaution to only introduce one new food at a time, and then give no other new food for two or three days. A new food may be offered once a day, starting with tiny amounts which are gradually increased. If a certain food does upset the baby, it should be withdrawn from the diet. Under no circumstances should a baby be forced to eat something he does not like; he might be allergic to it. Once a baby is accepting a range of foods, combinations of foods may be offered. This method of introducing new foods is particularly important if there are allergies in the family, or the baby has suffered from colic or other digestive disturbance.

Fluids other than milk, preferably plain boiled water, must be offered once mixed feeding has begun, particularly in hot weather or during illness. Babies sometimes develop constipation when weaning is initiated if they do not drink sufficient fluids. In some cases this leads to the development of an anal fissure, which results in painful defecation and increasing constipation. Giving the baby juice from stewed figs or prunes (available dried from health-food shops) will cause the stools to become very soft, allowing the fissure to heal.

As the baby gets older he will become more interested in the solids than the milk; he will then drink less and eat more. Eventually, when he is between six and nine months, he will be having three meals a day: breakfast, lunch and supper, and milk with his meals. Boiled water, or occasionally pure, unsweetened, very dilute fruit juice may be given between meals when he is thirsty. Fruit juices, even unsweetened ones, should never be given by bottle, however, as they remain in contact with the teeth for a long time and may lead to tooth decay. Babies under one year should drink about one pint of milk daily. Much more than this is probably not desirable as it may reduce the appetite for the iron-containing foods needed by infants who have been breast-fed, in order to avoid anaemia.

*meats at 4 mos*

Breast milk does not contain enough iron to satisfy nutritional needs after the first four to six months after birth, and iron-rich foods should be introduced first. Bottle-fed babies, while they are receiving a complete formula fortified with iron, obtain adequate iron. All meats are good sources of iron. Puréed or finely minced lamb, beef, veal, chicken, duck, turkey or liver may be introduced at four months. After six months pork may be introduced. Visible fat should be trimmed off the meat before serving. Ham, bacon, sausages, cured beef and tongue are not suitable foods for children as they are high in salt, preservatives and fat. Game (rabbit, pheasant, etc.) may be eaten provided that it does not contain lead shot.

*fish at 4 mos*

Fish is lower in iron than meat but still provides significant amounts and is a very nutritious, easy-to-digest food. It is a good idea to get the baby used to the taste at an early age. He can start off with filleted white fish such as plaice, sole, cod, whiting or haddock. When he is about a year old, fatty fish such as fresh herring, mackerel, trout or salmon can be introduced. Children should not eat shellfish; it can produce severe allergies, it concentrates toxins and if contaminated will result in violent stomach upsets. Fish which are canned, such as sardines, pilchards, tuna or salmon should be avoided, as canned food contains higher lead levels than the fresh equivalent. Tuna may also contain high levels of mercury.

*Veg*

Babies love vegetables, especially sweet-tasting ones such as carrots and parsnips. Other vegetables suitable for babies include peas, courgettes, potatoes, sweet potatoes, swedes, turnips, cabbage, cauliflower, Brussels sprouts, broccoli and many others. Spinach, however, is not suitable for babies under one year of age. It contains large quantities of nitrates which are converted to poisonous nitrites during storage. Most raw vegetables, other than bean sprouts, cress, etc., need not be given until a child is two years old, as they are digested too incompletely to be of value. Onions, leeks, sweetcorn, mushrooms and dried pulses (beans, peas and lentils) should be introduced with caution, as they frequently cause digestive problems.

*fruit*

Most fruit is excellent, providing it is fresh – not canned or frozen. It should be served raw. Ripe apples, pears and bananas are good to start off with, followed by peaches, apricots, plums, satsumas, pineapple, avocado pears, oranges, strawberries, raspberries and grapes. Grapes, apples and pears, etc., should be peeled at first, but the small seeds of raspberries and strawberries may be eaten. Citrus fruit or juice and strawberries should be introduced cautiously as these very frequently cause allergies in young babies. Symptoms include vomiting, diarrhoea, rashes, asthma, etc.

Fruit juices suitable for babies include very dilute pure orange or apple juice. These may be purchased in cartons from the milkman or any supermarket. Sugar is permitted in fruit juices and they need only be labelled 'sweetened' when more than 15g of sugar per litre has been added. Only those juices specifically labelled 'unsweetened' should be purchased. Apple juice may be bought as a concentrate from health-food shops.

Many mothers in the UK introduce cereals as the first food, but there is no evidence that these foods are nutritionally better than other foods. A baby's first cereal is usually rice. Wholegrain rice (brown rice) should be given in preference to 'baby' rice which is made from refined white rice. Some health-food shops sell brown rice flakes, ground rice or rice flour, which need little preparation. If these are not available, cooked brown rice may be made into a suitable consistency using a food blender, electric liquidizer or food processor.

Gluten-containing cereals – wheat, rye, barley, oats and buck-wheat – may be introduced when the baby is six months old, and so can corn (maize) and millet. Wholegrain flours or flakes (rice, barley, oats, corn and millet but not wheat and rye) cooked with water and mixed with breast milk, formula or cows' milk and some fresh apple, pear or banana, make a nourishing 'breakfast' for babies. Koh-koh is a highly nutritious unrefined baby food based on organically grown grain and pulses. It is suitable for babies over six months, and is available from some independent health food shops. Swiss Baby Cereal with no added sugar (a mixture of unprocessed cereals, dried fruits and nuts) may also be given.

An attempt is sometimes made to partially replace some of the nutrients lost during the processing of refined breakfast cereals, but even the most 'fortified' cereal can never be as good, nutritionally, as an unrefined cereal. Shredded Wheat (and Cubs) and Puffed Wheat are the only major brands of breakfast cereals that are both unrefined and free from added sugar or salt; the consistency of Shredded Wheat, however, makes this cereal unsuitable for babies under one year. Sugar or honey should never be added to cereals at the table.

Babies over six months may be given wholegrain breads, and pastas such as macaroni and spaghetti. When buying cereal products, the label must be read carefully and only 100 per cent wholegrain products purchased. Wholemeal bread may contain additives, including vitamin C as an improver, but it is not permitted to contain, in addition, the bleaches and other improvers used in brown (85–95 per cent extraction) and white flour. If possible, bread should be bought from health-food shops. It is often made with stoneground wholemeal flour from organically grown wheat and is usually free from additives.

'Spreads' suitable for babies over six months include sugar-free jam, unsweetened natural smooth peanut butter and other nut spreads, sunflower or sesame spread, Natex (low-salt) yeast extract, curd cheese, mashed ripe banana or ripe avocado. Honey, ordinary jam, marmalade, Marmite, chocolate spread, lemon curd and processed cheese and cheese spreads should be avoided.

Commercial rusks are not suitable for inclusion in a wholefood diet. They are made from white flour and are far too sweet to be recommended. As an alternative, wholegrain, salt-free, sugar-free, puffed rice cakes (from health-food shops) may be offered to babies over four months. Babies over six months enjoy rusks baked from wholemeal bread.

Eggs may be introduced when the baby is over six months old. If the baby refuses them, then they should be left until he is one year old. Free-range eggs are nutritionally superior to battery eggs and are available at shops displaying a yellow triangle. This certifies that the eggs are genuinely free-range.

Cows' milk and other dairy products may be introduced at six months. Government reports recommend that children under the age of five should drink whole milk rather than semi-skimmed or skimmed, as they usually obtain a substantial proportion of dietary energy from milk. Unsalted butter should be given rather than the salted variety. Any butter is preferable to soft or hard margarines. All pure vegetable oils from a specified source – excluding coconut and palm oil, which are highly saturated – may be eaten. Ideally they should be 'cold-pressed' as these have undergone little refining. Both butter and oils used for cooking or salads should be used sparingly.

Yoghurt is popular with babies. Only plain, unsweetened yoghurt is suitable, as most fruit varieties contain a lot of sugar – as much as four teaspoons in most popular brands – and other additives such as flavouring, colouring, modified starch, etc. Yoghurt is easy to make at home at a fraction of the cost of commercial ones. It keeps for up to two weeks under refrigeration.

Most babies like cheese; it is easier to digest if it is not cooked, but finely grated and stirred into the warm food. All cheese, other than cottage cheese, is high in fat and salt, so although it is a good source of protein, its consumption should be limited. The cheeses most suitable for young children include Cheddar and Cheshire-type cheeses, curd cheese, cream cheese, cottage cheese and most French cheeses. Processed cheese, smoked cheeses and cheese spread are best avoided as these contain additives. Nitrites are permitted in Edam and Gouda (from Holland) and some other cheeses.

Proprietary ice cream should be reserved for special occasions. A high percentage of the energy it provides comes from sugar and fat and it usually contains a variety of potentially harmful additives. Genuine dairy ice cream, free from artificial flavouring and colouring, is expensive but will do less harm to a baby's health. A nutritious ice cream may be made at home using fresh cream, eggs and orange juice. Home-made ice lollies may be enjoyed by babies towards the end of their first year. Frozen unsweetened diluted fruit juices or fresh fruit yoghurt make delicious ice lollies at very little cost. Peeled bananas cut in half and frozen on sticks are also popular.

Foods seasoned with herbs or a moderate amount of mild spices may be given to babies over six months. Any condiments which could cause discomfort, such as mustard or black pepper, should not be allowed and salt should never be added.

Many babies like to feed themselves. Finger foods suitable for babies under six months include peeled carrots, small cored peeled apples or puffed rice cakes. Care should be taken that the baby does not bite off large chunks of food which may make him choke. Babies over six months may be given pieces of cheese, home-made rusks, crusts of bread, chop bones, etc. A baby must never be left alone while he is eating.

## FOODS TO AVOID

The list of foods which babies should avoid, as they cannot possibly build health, includes many found in the supermarket. It is best to decide, preferably before weaning is started, whether time and effort is to be invested in helping the child to form healthy life-long food

# SUGGESTED WEEKLY MENU FOR BABIES BETWEEN FOUR AND SIX MONTHS

|  | Monday | Tuesday | Wednesday | Thursday | Friday | Saturday | Sunday |
|---|---|---|---|---|---|---|---|
| BREAKFAST | Ground rice and pear | Ground rice and banana | Ground rice and grapes | Ground rice and apple | Ground rice and plum | Ground rice and pear | Ground rice and banana |
| LUNCH | Carrot, potato and parsnip | Lamb and sweet potato | Chicken and green beans | Haddock and carrots | Brussels sprouts, swede and potato | Grilled lamb liver and broccoli | Beef broth (see recipes) |
|  | ½ teaspoon vegetable oil* | | ½ teaspoon vegetable oil | ½ teaspoon vegetable oil | ½ teaspoon vegetable oil | | |
| TEA | Apple | Plum | Avocado pear | Banana | Apple | Grapes | Peach |

NOTE: Most babies do not need to start solids until they are six months old, since unlimited breast milk plus a vitamin D supplement, or a complete infant formula, provide all the nutrients a baby requires up to this age. If solids are given, they should not be allowed to take the place of milk which is the most important part of the diet. A full milk feed should always be offered before the solid part of the meal, bearing in mind that a baby eating a lot of solids also needs extra water. The introduction of household cows' milk and gluten-containing cereals (wheat, rye, barley and oats), is best left until the baby is six months old.

* Oil should be polyunsaturated; e.g. safflower, soya, sunflower, corn or peanut. Cold-pressed oils are healthiest.

# SUGGESTED WEEKLY MENU FOR BABIES BETWEEN SIX AND TWELVE MONTHS

| | Monday | Tuesday | Wednesday | Thursday | Friday | Saturday | Sunday |
|---|---|---|---|---|---|---|---|
| **BREAKFAST** | Millet; Apple; Wholemeal bread*, butter, sugar-free jam; Milk | Porridge; Pear; Wholemeal bread, smooth peanut butter; Milk | Puffed Wheat; Satsuma; Wholemeal bread, sesame spread; Milk | Ground rice; Strawberries or raspberries; Wholemeal bread, peanut butter; Milk | Porridge; Melon; Wholemeal bread, curd cheese; Milk | Ground rice; Banana; Wholemeal bread, sunflower spread; Milk | Puffed Wheat; Plum; Wholemeal bread, sesame spread; Milk |
| **LUNCH** | Cottage pie* and cauliflower; Fresh fruit and natural yoghurt*; Apple juice | Boiled chicken and vegetable rice*; Orange ice cream* and fresh fruit; Water | Bean curd, broccoli, swede and parsley sauce*; Fresh fruit and natural yoghurt; Apple juice | Grilled cod*, mashed potato and peas; Fresh fruit and natural yoghurt; Orange juice | Barley and millet pilaff*; Fresh fruit and natural yoghurt; Apple juice | Vegetable bake* and mashed sweet potato; Winter warmer*; Orange juice | Roast beef, baked potato and brussels sprouts; Fresh fruit and natural yoghurt; Apple juice |
| **SUPPER** | Boiled egg, bread and butter; An orange; Milk | Avocado sandwich; Cheese, bean sprouts; Milk | Banana and cottage cheese sandwich; Milk | Cheese on toast; A tomato; Milk | Herring roes* on bread and butter; Blackberries; Milk | Scrambled egg*, bread and butter; Pear; Milk | Peanut butter and cress sandwich; Banana; Milk |

NOTE: Gluten-containing cereals (wheat, rye, barley and oats) may be introduced and so can diluted cows' milk (household) and other dairy produce. Citrus fruits and eggs may be added to the diet with caution. Food may be cut up small, grated, or mashed with a fork. Puréeing is no longer necessary. Milk is still the most important part of the diet, but the baby now needs a variety of foods in order to maintain optimum health.

SNACKS: rice cakes, home-made rusks*, raw carrot, raw celery, fresh fruit.

* See recipe section.

134 • A Good Start

habits in order to avoid disease. The foods children are allowed during their first years usually become their favourites throughout life. By giving a correct early diet many of the eating problems that commonly affect the older child may be avoided.

The following foods should not be given to babies under one year: smoked, cured, pickled or salted meat or fish (e.g. ham, some sausages, corned beef, bacon, cured tongue, kippers, smoked haddock, smoked roe), shellfish, spinach, adult canned food, Marmite, salt, sugar, alcohol, tea or coffee.

Foods to be strictly limited or avoided, if at all possible, include: all white flour products and most packaged cereals, sweets, chocolates, commercial ice cream, cakes, sweet biscuits, synthetic soft drinks (whole orange drink, lemonade, cola, etc.), honey, jam (except sugar-free varieties), processed cheese and cheese spreads, fried food and hydrogenated vegetable fats and oils (some margarines and many processed foods).

## PREPARING FOOD FOR A BABY

The preparation of food for a baby need not be time-consuming. When weaning is started – at about four months – the baby will only be eating teaspoonful amounts of foods, so it is not necessary to spend a lot of time cooking or shopping for him. There is no hard and fast rule that the baby must start on apple rather than banana, potato rather than swede, or chicken rather than lamb. If the baby seems to enjoy what he is given, and is not sick afterwards, all will be well.

Food is mashed or sieved to begin with, and kept semi-liquid by adding the cooking water, gradually building up to thicker, mashed foods and then to small pieces at about six or seven months. Babies do not need teeth in order to be able to masticate food, providing it is kept small. If the baby is fed for too long on puréed foods, he will probably reject lumpy food when it is finally introduced.

Preparing meals in bulk is the most efficient (but not the most nutritious) way of cooking for a young baby. All the ingredients are cooked in one saucepan; the foods which take longest to cook are added first and the quicker cooking ingredients later. A small amount of water is used so that very little remains after the food is cooked. The food is then sieved, mashed or blended with the cooking water. Excess cooking water should not be discarded as it contains many vitamins and minerals. Salt must not be added.

Food which is not eaten immediately is spooned into ice-cube trays or yoghurt pots, covered, and placed in the freezer as soon as it is cool. By preparing three or four main courses in advance and then freezing them, the baby will have a choice of menu on the days that fresh food has not been prepared. Frozen food containing meat or fish must be thawed, and then thoroughly reheated by boiling before serving.

Ripe fruit needs no cooking, but it should be peeled and cored. Soft fruit can be served to babies after mashing or sieving. Harder fruits, e.g. apples or pears, can be grated, using a fine-mesh grater. If fruit is to be cooked for special occasions, stewing conserves the most nutrients. Fruit should be stewed without sugar, if possible, and with the minimum of water. The water which clings to fruit after it has been washed is usually sufficient.

## COMMERCIAL BABY FOODS

Provided a mother understands the basics of nutrition and is prepared to spend a little time in the kitchen, she need never have to buy the expensive ready-prepared commercial baby foods. Many mothers think – most likely as a result of forceful advertising – that a baby's health, growth and well-being depend on the progression from formula or breast milk to jars, packets and cans especially prepared for them. Commercial baby foods (with a very few exceptions) have no part to play in a wholefood diet and contribute to the development in later life of such Western diseases as heart disease, high blood pressure, diabetes and obesity.

Preparing the baby's food from the raw ingredients is more time-consuming than buying it ready prepared, but this is a small sacrifice to make when the advantages it offers the child in terms of superior health are considered. It is very easy to wean a baby on to a mixed diet without ever having to resort to commercial weaning foods, even when travelling. Such babies invariably enjoy good health and a vigorous appearance, and readily accept the transition from weaning foods to food that the family is eating without the fuss commonly seen among children raised on highly processed food.

To understand why most commercial baby foods are not suitable for inclusion in a wholefood diet, it is necessary to examine what is in them and how they are prepared. Commercial baby foods contain a wide range of ingredients including meats, cereals, dairy products, vegetables and fruits. This means that mothers buying these products can easily select for their babies what is traditionally considered in the Western world to be a 'balanced' diet, especially since this task is simplified by the classification of products into breakfasts, dinners and desserts.

All the commonly eaten flours or cereals are used in weaning foods. These flours are usually refined, however, which means that the bran and the germ have been removed, and with them valuable nutrients. Baby foods often contain modified starches, such as modified cornflour, a virtually pure starch. Modified starches may supply 10–32 per cent of the energy content of strained and junior dinners, desserts and fruits. Purified starch (a highly refined carbohydrate) provides 'empty' calories, failing, like sugar, to bring with it the complement of vitamins, minerals and proteins that is needed to carry on the metabolism that it could energize.

Modified starch contains phosphates. If a baby eats food containing added phosphate (an essential mineral), he will consume larger amounts than would be the case if his diet consisted of unprocessed foods. There are indications that an excessive daily intake of phosphate can lead to the premature cessation of bone growth in children, with a consequent significant reduction in adult height.

Optional ingredients in baby foods include sugar and salt. Salt is usually added to weaning foods during manufacture to suit the palate of the mother rather than the baby, based on the theory that if none is added, the mother will herself add an uncontrolled amount. A young baby's kidneys cannot cope with too much salt, and salt intake throughout life, and particularly for a period in infancy, may influence adult blood pressure.

Of the prepared foods currently available, there is generally no added salt in strained fruits and juices; 0.4–0.6 per cent is added to strained meats, dinners and soups; less than 0.4 per cent is added to desserts and 1 per cent to cereal products. Many well-known brands of baby food claim to contain no added salt. This is not always accurate, however, since the ingredients which make up the meals may contain salt. Meals containing cheese, bacon or sausage for example, will contain salt, since salt is always added to these foods during their manufacture.

There have been suggestions that the introduction at an early age of foods sweetened with sucrose or other sugars may establish a preference for sweet foods. The consumption of sweet foods causes dental decay and is associated with many other diseases. Due to inadequate labelling, however, it is impossible to ascertain exactly how much sugar is present in baby foods. Where nutritional analyses are available – either on the label or from the manufacturer – it is customary to give details of the total carbohydrate present in foods. This carbohydrate includes both the beneficial complex type found in grains, beans and peas and also the simple carbohydrates (sugars). It does not distinguish between them.

Many babies are totally dependent on specially prepared weaning foods for their nutrition. Although almost every manufactured weaning food contains added nutrients to replace losses which occur through processing, they can never be expected to contain all the nutrients that were present in the unprocessed food. This is particularly true for the lesser known essential nutrients, such as the more obscure B vitamins or trace elements. Most baby meals are pre-cooked and only need reheating if necessary, but mothers frequently 'cook' these meals again, with the result that weaning foods often suffer from proportionately greater nutrient losses than fresh home-prepared food.

Rusks and fruit syrups complete the range of foods specially marketed for babies and young children. Rusks are prepared from refined cereal, sugar, fat, skimmed milk, added vitamins and various other ingredients. Because of consumer (mothers') demand for less sweet food, 'low-sugar' rusks are now extensively marketed. For most people, this statement implies that the product contains very little sugar. In fact, although all 'low-sugar' rusks contain less sugar than their predecessors, they usually contain more sugar, gram for gram, than doughnuts, currant buns or plain digestive biscuits. Furthermore, the percentage of sugar they claim to contain only represents the sucrose (table sugar) content and ignores the glucose and other sugars that are frequently present. The labelling on a leading brand of rusks, for example, claims that they contain 18 per cent sugar (sucrose); but if the other sugars are included, this percentage rises to 22.3 per cent.

Babies do not have a physiological need for sugar, and sugar consumption has been shown to be a direct cause of tooth decay. It does not matter whether the sugar is sucrose, glucose, fructose or maltose; they are all bad for the teeth. The newly erupting teeth of a young baby are particularly vulnerable to decay.

Fruit syrups (Baby Ribena, etc.) are highly sweetened, concentrated fruit juices providing supplementary vitamin C. They may cause tooth decay, particularly when given by bottle or when the daily dosage as specified on the label is exceeded. Fruit syrups are sometimes preserved with sulphur-containing preservatives. These are potentially toxic and are best avoided. Some syrups also contain salt (sodium chloride). If the baby is thirsty between meals, he should be offered water. Fresh fruit will provide ample vitamin C.

Sterile bottles of unsweetened fruit juice with added vitamin C, marketed by baby-food manufacturers, need never be purchased. They are very expensive and offer little advantage over 'adult' pure juices, which are much cheaper.

## DO CHILDREN NEED NUTRITIONAL SUPPLEMENTS?

If the mother is breast-feeding and exposes her baby every day to the sun, he may not need supplements provided she is eating an excellent diet. A bottle-fed baby who is given artificial feeds prepared from a proprietary infant formula containing a full complement of vitamins and minerals will not need a supplement.

When mixed feeding is introduced, and especially if, after the age of six months, the baby begins to drink household cows' milk, the possibility of vitamin deficiency is greater. Nearly all refined foods marketed for infants and toddlers are enriched with vitamins, and most household diets are thought to contain adequate amounts of all vitamins, except D. There may be some babies, however, who are offered a diet containing insufficient vitamins, or who are reluctant to consume enough of the necessary vitamin-containing foods. There is also the possibility of vitamin D deficiency, due to insufficient sunlight reaching bare skin, especially in the winter months.

Recent scientific evidence has shown that a high-fibre diet will increase vitamin D requirements, particularly if the consumption of animal foods such as meat, fish and eggs is reduced. Babies weaned on to a wholefood diet, especially a vegetarian one, are therefore particularly at risk of vitamin D deficiency.

Although a baby is unlikely to get overt rickets if not given a vitamin D supplement, he may grow up with some of the milder manifestations of vitamin D deficiency. These include frequent respiratory infections, a flat, narrow chest, poor jaw development, crooked, overcrowded teeth, a receding or bulging forehead, a narrow or misshapen face and eyes too close together.

Children's Vitamin Drops (available from child health clinics) containing vitamins A, C and D, or a suitable amount of a proprietary preparation of vitamin D, should be given to a child during the entire growth period for optimum health, starting when a breast-fed baby is one month old. If a baby is bottle-fed, however, with a complete infant formula containing added vitamins A and D, dietary supplementation may be initiated when weaning is begun; but the full dose should only be given when infant formula is no longer drunk.

Vitamins A and D are fat-soluble and are stored in the body fat, so although it is important that the child has an optimal daily intake, too much is dangerous. The instructions must be carefully read and the dose never exceeded. Only one supplement of vitamin D should be given at one time. A very rich natural source of vitamins A and D, which can be given when the baby is six months old, is fish-liver oil, and this used to be the recommended nutritional supplement for children until it was superseded by synthetic water-soluble preparations.

Fish-liver oils are preferable to the synthetic water-soluble vitamins since they retain their potency longer and are a good source of iodine. Furthermore, since the water-soluble preparations of vitamin A are absorbed far more rapidly than the fish-liver oils, they have caused most of the cases of vitamin A toxicity resulting from overdosage. Fish-liver oil should be given from a bottle rather than as capsules as young children cannot absorb the oil from these well. A brand should be chosen which also contains vitamin E, since polyunsaturated oils dramatically increase the need for this vitamin. The dose should be given after a meal containing fat.

The use of multivitamin and mineral supplements is usually only necessary when the child is ill enough to prevent him from eating properly for more than a few days. When looking for a suitable preparation, labels must be carefully read to make sure that it is recommended for children.

## THE WORKING MOTHER

Many mothers go back to work after having a baby, either for financial reasons or because they do not find looking after children sufficiently fulfilling. Some mothers are fortunate enough to have relatives living near by who are prepared to look after their children for them while they go out to work. Other mothers send their children to a child-minder. The most expensive, but most satisfactory arrangement, however, is to employ a daily or live-in nanny or mother's help to look after the child at home.

The most important decision which working mothers must make, is when to go back to work. Exclusive breast-feeding plays a very important role in good child nutrition as it lays the foundations upon which superior health is built. Unless it is absolutely necessary, it is inadvisable to go back to work full-time until a breast-fed baby is at least six months old. (The mother should be able to get maternity leave until then.) This is because the majority of breast-fed babies will have to be partially or totally formula fed when the mother returns to work, and this will inevitably increase the risk of the baby developing allergies such as eczema or asthma and also lower his immunity to infection.

Expressing breast milk for a child-minder or nanny to give the baby is possible, but this only works well if the mother is not going to be out for more than one feed a day. It also requires a lot of willpower and perseverance, as the mother may need to express milk while at work for her baby to drink the next day or to stimulate the milk supply or to relieve discomfort. Expressed milk must be put into a sterile container and refrigerated if it is to be kept.

Once a baby has started solids, he will be unlikely to be fed on wholefoods if he is looked after by a child-minder, unless the mother is prepared to make the baby's meals before work and give them to the child-minder to warm up. As soon as the child is old enough to know what is going on, however, he will expect to eat what the other children are eating. Furthermore, it will be impossible to stop the child-minder giving the child an occasional sweet to stop him crying, for example. The same applies to day-nurseries; here one cannot dictate what the child is going to eat, as the meals are mass-produced.

It is therefore apparent that working outside the home and good child nutrition are unlikely to be compatible unless the child can be looked after at home. This does not mean that any plans for raising the child on a healthy diet will have to be abandoned – just scaled down.

A compromise can probably be reached with the child-minder or day-nursery supervisor, in which the mother provides some of her child's food or drink, such as puffed brown rice cakes, dried fruit, an apple or diluted fruit juice, which he can be given at times when the other children are having sweets, biscuits or sweetened soft drinks.

Raising a child on a healthy diet is not easy when one has to contend with powerful advertising, the differing attitudes of other people and the natural contrariness of children. But when the mother is working it becomes even more difficult and she will need all the determination she can muster in order to succeed.

# FEEDING THE OVER-ONES

Once mixed feeding is established, it is no longer necessary to prepare food specially for the baby, unless it is more convenient to do so. He can join in meals with the rest of the family provided they are also eating wholefoods. Many parents will therefore need to make substantial changes to their diets in the interests of their children's health.

## THE DAILY ROUTINE

By the time a baby reaches his first birthday, he should be eating three meals a day: breakfast, lunch and supper. Breakfast between 7 and 9 a.m., lunch between 12 and 2 p.m. and supper between 4.30 and 6.30 p.m. Young children, like adults, do not need two large cooked meals a day and will thrive on one main meal, eaten either at midday or in the evening. Ideally this meal should be served at lunch-time, especially if the child goes to bed early, since going to sleep straight after a large meal may cause digestive upsets.

The traditional (although declining in popularity) British breakfast of fried egg, bacon, sausage, tomato and white bread and butter is not a habit for young children to adopt. A large proportion of the energy provided by this type of meal comes from fat, and the consumption of saturated fats (butter, animal fat, hard margarine, etc.) has been shown to be an important contributory factor in the development of heart disease. This type of breakfast also contains salt, preservatives, refined cereals and often colouring.

A healthy breakfast for the under-fives includes a wholegrain cereal, such as sugar-free muesli, porridge, Puffed Wheat, Cubs or Shredded Wheat, with milk. Muesli may be home-made or purchased ready mixed. It may, however, cause intestinal irritability or diarrhoea in young children. To make it more digestible, it should be ground up using a food processor or liquidizer, soaked in milk and left in the fridge overnight. Alternatively, Swiss Baby Cereal with no added sugar is available from leading chemists, health-food shops and some supermarkets.

Porridge made with fresh oatmeal or oatflakes, without added sugar or salt, is very nutritious. Sweetened 'instant' porridge should be avoided. Almost all the commercial breakfast cereals, with a few exceptions, are refined and contain added sugar and salt. They are not suitable for inclusion in a wholefood diet. Fresh or dried fruit, but never sugar, syrup or honey, may be added to cereals at the table.

Bread should be wholemeal. Brown bread is made from 85 per cent extraction flour and contains 40 per cent less dietary fibre than wholemeal bread. If wholemeal bread is not well tolerated then whole rye bread or rye crispbread (Ryvita) are good substitutes. Bread may be spread with unsweetened natural peanut butter, sesame spread, sunflower spread, a little butter and sugar-free jam or occasionally low-salt Natex savoury spread. Bread is preferable to toast as it is more nutritious, and burnt or browned foods are potential carcinogens. Some fresh fruit should be included in a baby's breakfast. It provides vitamin C, which increases the absorption of iron from cereal foods.

The main meal of the day should include a small portion of meat, white or fatty fish, eggs, cheese, soya, or grains and pulses and a green or yellow vegetable. If the child is going to be eating the same food as the rest of the family, then salt should not be added to the cooking pot. Alternatively the child's portion may be removed before adding seasoning.

The 'quickest' healthy dessert is natural, unsweetened yoghurt and fresh fruit. Occasionally, other desserts free from sugar or honey may be given. Processed gelatine desserts, sweetened commercial yoghurts, jellies and steamed puddings should be avoided. These are health-destroying foods and are high in anti-nutrients such as sugar.

Supper need only be a light, easy-to-prepare meal, consisting of eggs, occasionally cheese, wholemeal bread and butter, fresh unsalted nuts or nut butter, sunflower or pumpkin seeds, fresh fruit and some finely grated raw vegetables such as carrot, lettuce, chicory, tomato, bean sprouts or cress for younger children, and

radish, celery, cucumber or spinach for the older ones. Raw
vegetables may be lightly dressed with a little cold-pressed polyunsaturated vegetable oil, some lemon juice and yoghurt. Polyunsaturated oils should ideally only be used for salads or cold dishes
as they may form harmful substances when heated. Olive oil (a
monounsaturated oil) may be used for shallow frying as it is more
stable when heated than the polyunsaturated oils.

Children between one and five only require between 280 and
425 ml (½ and ¾ pt) of milk daily, as it should now be regarded as a
supplement to solid food rather than a replacement for it. It should
be offered as a drink with breakfast and supper. Diluted, unsweetened, fresh, pure fruit juices, such as apple or orange, should be
reserved for mealtimes – lunchtime is ideal – as they may cause
tooth decay if drunk frequently between meals. Fresh fruit juices,
but not squashes or fruit drinks, are very high in potassium. Potassium acts to protect against the effect of a high salt intake and so
limits the development of high blood pressure. Synthetic fruit
drinks, cola and fizzy drinks are to be strictly avoided as they are
essentially solutions of chemicals. Tea, coffee and alcohol must
never be given, no matter how dilute they are.

## SNACK FOODS

There are few, if any, children (or adults for that matter) who do not
regularly eat between meals, and snack foods often make a significant contribution to the diet. What the child is offered in the way of
snacks is therefore just as important as what he is eating at mealtimes, and an effort should be made to ensure that these foods are as
nutritious and health-promoting as possible. Snacks may consist of
a few unsalted, broken nuts or seeds, a piece of fruit, some cheese,
dried fruit or a wholegrain biscuit or crispbread.

Up to a certain age, children are generally unaware of the existence of junk foods. If a three-year-old child has been accustomed to
wholefoods, then healthy likes and dislikes are established. It is only
later on that a child asks for junk foods, e.g. crisps and ice lollies as
advertised on TV or eaten by playmates. Parents should not be
influenced by ideas such as 'all children eat sweets' or 'he mustn't
feel different from other children'. One's own child is someone
special who needs protection from commercial exploitation and
the 'tasty toxins' – sweets, chocolates, ice lollies, crisps and cola

# SUGGESTED WEEKLY MENU FOR CHILDREN BETWEEN ONE AND FIVE YEARS

| | Monday | Tuesday | Wednesday | Thursday | Friday | Saturday | Sunday |
|---|---|---|---|---|---|---|---|
| **BREAKFAST** | Muesli* Satsuma Bread and peanut butter Milk | Porridge Pear Bread, butter and sugar-free jam Milk | Shredded Wheat Grapes Bread and sesame spread Milk | Muesli Orange Ryvita and curd cheese Milk | Porridge Plum Bread and sunflower spread Milk | Muesli Apple Bread and peanut butter Milk | Puffed Wheat Banana Bread, butter and sugar-free jam Milk |
| **LUNCH** | Vegetable and bean hotpot with cheese sauce* Fresh fruit and natural yoghurt Apple juice | Grilled herring*, mashed potato and baked beans* Fresh fruit and natural yoghurt Orange juice | Spaghetti bolognese* Hawaiian cocktail* Apple juice | Beef and vegetable stew* Fresh fruit and natural yoghurt Apple juice | Grilled haddock, mashed potato and swede Fresh fruit and natural yoghurt Apple juice | Barley and bean casserole* Apple snow* Orange juice | Roast lamb, roast potatoes and cabbage Orange surprise* Apple juice |
| **SUPPER** | Chopped liver* sand- wich Mixed salad* Fruit Milk | Cheesy baked potato* and bean sprouts Fruit Milk | Wholewheat pancakes and sugar-free jam Fruit Milk | Avocado and tomato sand- wich Fruit Milk | Cheese on toast Mixed salad Fruit Milk | Boiled egg, toast and butter Fruit Milk | Peanut butter and cress sandwich Fruit Milk |

NOTE: From the second year onwards the growth of the child slows down. Milk should now be regarded as a supplement to food, rather than instead of food – an average amount of 280–425 ml (½–¾ pt) per day is quite sufficient. After his first birthday he can start to join in family meals, but his salt intake should be limited by not adding it to his food.

SNACKS: fresh fruit, dried fruit (in moderation), cheese, wholemeal crispbread with butter.

* See recipe section.

drinks – with their sugar, salt, fat and stimulants. An informed mother who loves her children enough not to want to see them suffer, simply does not bring such junk foods into the house.

One big snack is better than a lot of little snacks, since the more often snacks containing carbohydrate (sugar or starch) are eaten – even wholefood ones – the greater the risk of tooth decay. Snacks must be strictly limited, however, if the child lacks appetite at mealtimes. For a young child without pocket money, this should not be too difficult.

## SWITCHING TO A WHOLEFOOD DIET

Ideally, a child should be weaned from the breast on to a wholefood diet. It is never too late, however, for a child to switch from a refined diet to an unrefined one. Any improvement in diet at any age will result in better health. Furthermore, some of the damage caused by a poor diet can be reversed, though by how much will depend on the child's age. The younger he is, the greater the potential for improvement will be.

Changing a child's eating habits should be done slowly. New foods should be introduced gradually while continuing the old regime. It is best to start replacing between-meal snacks with wholefoods, and then slowly and subtly to effect changes in the child's meals. If, for example, the child's breakfast previously consisted of a bowl of sugar-coated Frosties, white bread and a glass of chocolate-flavoured milk, one can begin by replacing the white bread with wholemeal bread and introducing a piece of fruit. A small amount of muesli may then be added to his cereal and the quantity increased each day until eventually he is eating muesli rather than sugary, refined cereals. If he is old enough to object to these 'new' foods, it may be explained that by eating these healthy foods he will get fewer coughs and colds, tummy-aches, toothaches, etc. He should be reminded of the times when he has been ill.

If lunch is usually breaded fish and chips with tomato ketchup, hamburger and canned baked beans, corned beef and spaghetti hoops, or similar, then the child should be given these foods but in smaller quantities, together with a side dish of grated carrots, celery, cucumber, avocado pear, tomato, beetroot or bean sprouts with a little salad dressing. Instead of deep frying his food, it should be sautéed, grilled, steamed or boiled. Gradually, the fish-fingers and hamburgers may be replaced with unbreaded fish, chicken, lean meat or vegetarian dishes, and the vegetables cooked for a shorter time in a very small amount of water. Sugar-free (but not salt-free) tomato ketchup is available from health-food shops and may be substituted for highly sweetened ketchup. Natural, unsweetened yoghurt with fresh fruit added should be introduced as dessert, and sugary packet desserts no longer served.

For supper, boiled or scrambled eggs should replace fried eggs. Home-made baked beans made from dried haricot beans and fresh tomatoes should be served instead of canned beans, hard margarine and jam replaced with unsalted butter and sugar-free jam, and sweetened artificially saturated peanut butter replaced with natural sugar-free peanut butter. Each day the quantity of nutritious foods served to the child should be increased and the undesirable foods reduced.

Children under the age of two are unlikely to offer much resistance to the switch to a wholefood diet, if carried out gradually. For older children, however, far more cunning and persuasion will be needed if the changeover is to remain untraumatic. Perhaps the most important point to remember is that if children are allowed no snacks between meals – wholefood or otherwise – then they will be hungry enough to eat whatever is put in front of them at mealtimes.

## EATING PROBLEMS

All normal children go through phases, particularly in the second year, in which they become 'hunger strikers', refusing all food, according to their parents. Other children become finicky eaters, often existing on a bizarre diet. This affects as many as 30 per cent of four-year-olds, when the peak incidence is reached. Parents often cajole, bully, bribe and even batter their children to eat, turning mealtimes into a battlefield.

The amount of food which small children consume varies widely, but certainly many of them manage to thrive on what seems very little to adult eyes. If a child has little appetite it is extremely difficult not to worry, but parental anxiety is nearly always the cause of food faddishness. The child refuses his lunch, the parent fusses and worries, he does it again and the parent becomes even more attentive. A child quickly learns, certainly before his second birthday, that a good way of getting attention is by refusing his meals. Sometimes he may even be given 'treats' such as ice cream or biscuits, because the parent is afraid that he may be harmed by not eating enough.

Not all children who refuse to eat are going through fads. An ill or sickening child goes off his food and then it is not difficult to understand the reason for his lack of appetite. In these circumstances a child should not be forced to eat. Less obvious illnesses such as mild glandular fever or undiagnosed urinary infections may also reduce a child's appetite, and medical advice should therefore always be sought. Cystic fibrosis, coeliac disease and food allergy can cause eating difficulties, but these are nearly always diagnosed because there are other problems, too, which occur at a younger age. As a general rule, if the child is active, growing and happy (other than at mealtimes) there is unlikely to be anything physically wrong with him.

Having excluded ill health, the best treatment for food faddishness and meal refusal is firstly to make sure the child maintains his appetite. If he has had crisps, ice cream, chocolate, sweets, orange squash or cola, etc., between meals, he cannot be expected to sit at the table with enthusiasm and his negative behaviour would be justified. These junk foods are classified as such because although they are tasty they are nutritionally empty. Wholefood snacks such as nuts, fruit or milk can also blunt the appetite and should only be allowed if the child eats his meals.

When a child refuses his meal it pays to make as little fuss as possible. An occasional missed meal certainly does no harm. If he refuses to eat certain foods, an effort should be made to respect his wishes. Every child dislikes a few things. If he does not like cabbage, for example, then he may be offered another green vegetable such as broccoli or beans. A few weeks later he will probably have forgotten that he does not like cabbage and eat it with enthusiasm. The same principle may be used with other food groups. If he does not like beef then he may be offered lamb, if carrots are not in favour then another red or yellow vegetable such as swede or tomatoes are alternatives.

Some children love sauces, such as cheese or parsley sauce, and these may be served with the foods they are not so keen on. Presentation of food is very important. Just as adults like the food on their plates to look attractive, so do children. The meat, potatoes and vegetables should not all be mixed together but put separately on the plate. It is better to serve too little food and then offer seconds, than offer too much, which can be very offputting to a child.

If the child does not finish everything that is on his plate, he should not be forced to do so. Children who have been trained always to leave the plate clean frequently become obese adults, as they do not stop eating when they are no longer hungry, but keep eating until the plate is empty. As adults, they are also likely to feel guilty about throwing food away and so eat other people's leftovers, another habit which often leads to unwanted weight gain.

Sometimes children refuse to eat the main course but want the dessert. It certainly does no harm to let the child have his dessert first occasionally, as long as it is highly nutritious – a small amount of natural, unsweetened yoghurt and some fresh fruit, for example. It is when the dessert consists of sweetened yoghurt, jelly, a pudding, etc., rich in 'empty' calories, that health problems arise.

Consistency of approach is very important when dealing with eating problems. The above management should give results within a week or two, although sometimes it is necessary to persevere for several weeks.

## THE SICK CHILD

During active infections such as colds, chickenpox, German measles, measles or tonsillitis, a baby's requirement for almost every nutrient rises. The body's tissue stores are used to provide the immune system with needed protein, vitamins, and minerals to fight the infection. At the same time, the digestion and absorption of all nutrients decreases and losses in perspiration, urine and faeces soar.

A child's lack of appetite may result in his diet becoming drastically inadequate at the very time his nutritional needs are greatest. Frequently he may be offered only juice or toast, or perhaps tempted with foods having no nutritional value. Too much refined, sweet or fatty food won't help the child to get better and may make him constipated. The malnutrition which originally invited his infection becomes increasingly more severe as he develops deficiencies of protein, vitamins A, C, E, all the B vitamins and many minerals; thus one infection usually follows another.

During an acute infection, the diet should include easily digestible foods rich in protein and energy. Breast milk, formula, egg yolks and chicken soup are all excellent. It is imperative that the child drinks plenty of fluids to replace losses incurred through vomiting, diarrhoea or perspiration. Fruit juices may be given instead of water, but soft drinks are definitely out and so are junk foods. Nutritional supplements are particularly important when a child is sick, so if the child is no longer being given Children's Vitamin Drops or cod-liver oil, etc., now is the time to reintroduce them.

Presenting ordinary food in a special way, such as mashed potato and vegetables in the form of a face, may encourage the child to eat. Curly straws, fancy paper cups and plates and similar innovations may also encourage him to take the fluids and nourishment he needs.

# 11   🥐 · 🍅 · 🥕 · 🍎 · 🐟 · 🌶

# VEGETARIAN DIETS

Vegetarians do not eat flesh foods in any form, but the majority consume some animal products, such as milk, cheese and eggs. In general, the nutritional value of a good vegetarian diet is very similar to a non-vegetarian one. Mothers who intend to raise their babies as vegetarians should have a very good knowledge of nutrition in order to select a suitable diet for them. They must also be particularly vigilant in avoiding junk foods.

Vegans (strict vegetarians) do not eat either flesh foods or any animal products. Although man's nutrient requirements, with the exception of vitamin $B_{12}$, can be met by a diet composed entirely of plant foods, to do so it must be carefully planned, using a wide selection of highly nutritious foods. A mixture of plant proteins will provide adequate protein of good quality, but special care is needed to ensure that sufficient energy (calories), calcium, iron, riboflavin, vitamin $B_{12}$ and vitamin D are also available. If supplementary vitamin $B_{12}$ is not provided for vegans, then megaloblastic anaemia almost always develops. The disease causes pallor and tiredness, and results in the degeneration of the nervous system.

Vegetarianism offers many health benefits. Childhood obesity is virtually unknown among vegetarians, and because no meat and often no dairy products are eaten, levels of cholesterol are very low. This substantially reduces the risk of heart and blood vessel disease in later life. Gout and cancer of the bowel are extremely rare, with much higher rates being observed in meat eaters. On the negative side, although vegetarian diets are nutritionally adequate for adults, they may not be completely suitable for rapidly growing infants and young children. This is especially true for a vegan diet which is often lacking in calcium and energy.

## THE VEGETARIAN CHILD'S DIET

Most vegetarian and vegan babies are breast-fed, and their nutritional requirements can usually be met provided that they are exposed to sunlight and the mother takes a supplement of vitamin $B_{12}$. As a precaution against vitamin deficiency, however, all babies from the age of one month must be given vitamins A, C and D (drops or fortified cod-liver oil) at least until the age of five. Vegan babies should also be given a vitamin $B_{12}$ supplement after weaning.

Breast-feeding should carry on as long as possible. If the mother is not able to breast-feed, the baby may be bottle-fed with a complete infant formula based on cows' milk. Vegan babies, who are not allowed cows' milk, must have a soya-based milk substitute which they continue to drink throughout the whole growth period. It is very important that the product chosen is suitable as the sole source of nourishment for young babies. Examples are Formula S Soya Food, Pro Sobee and Wysoy. Some other soya-based milk substitutes may not meet the requirements of either young babies or toddlers and pre-school children. When weaning is initiated, a healthy diet will need to include a mixture of grains, beans, peas, lentils, nuts and seeds, vegetables and fruit. Eggs and dairy products are also usually eaten.

### Grains

Grains are the seeds of grasses, the best known being rice, oats, wheat, barley and rye. Whole grains are preferable to milled or processed grains because B vitamins, fibre, iron and vitamin E are lost during the milling process.

If properly prepared, grains can be fed as one of the baby's first foods. Grains should be introduced in the following order: first brown rice, then barley and millet, followed by oats and maize and finally wheat, the hardest of grains to digest and the one most likely to cause allergies, particularly in babies under six months of age. Grains must be thoroughly cooked and ground into a smooth paste before serving to a baby.

Grains may be combined with pulses or milk products for good-quality protein. Some grains may also be served with some seeds, for example bread with sesame or sunflower-seed spreads and rice with sesame seeds, to form complete protein. Complementary proteins must be eaten together at the same meal (see Protein, pp. 21–4).

## Pulses

Pulses – peas, beans and lentils – are also seeds, but are found within plant pods. They include soya beans, chick peas, kidney beans, mung beans, pinto beans, black-eye beans, split peas and lentils. Pulses are harder to digest than grains and so should not be given to a baby until he is eight or nine months old. All pulses, except for split red lentils, split peas and black-eye beans, should be soaked overnight and drained, and they must all be boiled for at least ten minutes before leaving them to simmer until they are soft (up to four hours). They should be blended and sieved to remove the husks, which are hard to digest.

Some pulses are processed in order to make them more digestible. Tofu (soya bean curd) is a highly digestible processed form of soya beans. Soya beans have the highest protein content of all the pulses and are rich in iron. They should therefore form a significant part of the vegetarian diet. Tofu should be kept as fresh as possible by storing it in the refrigerator under water which is changed periodically. Tofu can be used without cooking for salad dressings and dips. It can be mashed, fried, made into 'burgers', scrambled, put into soups, used as a replacement for cheese or meat in lasagne, pizza, etc., and also in cheesecake and puddings. Other soya products include soya milk and yoghurt. Soya beans are often the basis of commercial meatless protein foods.

## Bean sprouts

Pulses, like almost any seed, can be sprouted. Not all sprouts taste good, however, or are even edible. The best seeds to sprout are alfalfa, lentil, mung bean, soya bean, sunflower and wheat. Sprouts contain more nutrients than unsprouted beans and seeds, and in some cases these nutrients are more easily digestible. Furthermore, vitamin C is actually created while the seed is sprouting. Sprouts are a convenient source of fresh vegetables since they can be grown quickly at home.

To grow bean sprouts, the pulses or seeds are washed and soaked overnight to soften. The next day the water, which is full of nutrients, is poured off into another jar and used for cooking. The seeds are rinsed and drained. The jar is then covered with a paper towel and rubber band, or fine screen to help conserve moisture but to allow fresh air in, so the beans do not rot. The jar is tilted slightly and put in a warm, dark place. The seeds are rinsed about three times daily.

Sprouts take from two to six days to reach the desired length. On the last day, the jar is brought out of the dark and placed in a sunny spot until the leaves turn green. The sprouts are given one final rinse. Everything in the jar may be eaten. Sprouts can be ground up for young babies, put into salads, or combined with other vegetables in stir-fry dishes and casseroles.

## Nuts and seeds

Nuts and sesame, sunflower and pumpkin seeds have a similar nutritional value. They are rich sources of fat, protein, fibre and some minerals. Whole nuts and seeds cannot be digested by babies, but delicious nut and seed 'milks' can be made by soaking them overnight and then blending them with the soaking water. Any small pieces may be removed by straining. By grinding nuts and seeds a paste may be obtained. Nuts and seeds should be purchased in small quantities as they go rancid quickly, and stored either in the refrigerator or in a cool spot.

Nut and seed 'milks' can be given to babies when weaning is started. Pastes can be introduced at eight to ten months, but whole nuts and seeds should not be given until the child is able to chew well, between two and three.

## Vegetables

Vegetables are rich in vitamins, minerals and fibre. Dark green leaves contain the most nutrients. All fresh vegetables are sources of vitamin C, but it rapidly declines during storage, cooking and processing. Green and yellow/orange vegetables (carrots) are sources of vitamin A (as carotene). Other root vegetables and white vegetables contain none. Vegetables contain a small amount of protein and vitamin E, but are not good sources of B vitamins apart from folic acid. Dark green vegetables are rich in iron and calcium, but they are poorly absorbed. Spinach is not suitable for babies under one year and only leaves in good condition should be given to older children.

Care should be taken to buy crisp, fresh vegetables and these should be stored in a refrigerator until needed. Vegetables should be washed and cut up just before cooking and cooked in as little boiling water as possible. Vegetables and grains should be cooked in the same saucepan until all the cooking water is absorbed. If vegetables are cooked separately, the water should be used for cooking pulses and grains.

**Dairy products and eggs**

Dairy products – milk, yoghurt, cheese and butter, and also eggs – are rich in protein, vitamin $B_{12}$, calcium and other B vitamins and minerals. As these replace meat and fish in the diet, they should be eaten frequently. Vegan children do not eat these animal foods and alternatives such as soya products must be provided.

# SPECIAL OCCASIONS

Celebration meals are part of everyone's life, but for children brought up on wholefoods this often means having to eat health-destroying highly refined foods. With a bit of forward planning, however, these occasions can be enjoyed without having to depart too radically from a wholefood diet.

### BIRTHDAY PARTIES

Few children reach school age without having been to a birthday party. All too often the party menu reads like a list of all the foods that young children should most avoid: sugar in various forms (icing, confectionery, bakery products, soft drinks and jelly), artificial colourings (soft drinks, jelly, cakes, biscuits and icing), refined flour (white bread, pastry, cakes and biscuits), preservatives (soft drinks and sausages), drugs (caffeine in cola drinks) and salt (savoury snacks).

Luckily, children do not usually eat much at parties, yet the sight of well-meaning mothers imploring their offspring to eat more 'rubbish', seemingly unaware of the harm they are doing them, is horrifying. Although the effects are most serious in the allergic child, who may suffer an immediate unpleasant reaction, an otherwise healthy child will still be affected; by damage to his teeth, by reaction to noxious stimulants (caffeine) and by the loss from his body of valuable vitamins and minerals that are used up in the metabolism of sugar. It takes willpower on the part of parents to be different from other parents and to offer party fare that is nutritious, rather than the usual junk food, which may look more attractive.

Tea parties for small children should not be too ambitious, as generally more food remains on plates (or on the floor) than is actually eaten. Sandwiches made with wholemeal bread are nutritious, cheap and filling, and if a little ingenuity is used in their preparation and presentation, most children will eat them, even if there are cakes and biscuits on the table. Fillings should either be fresh or contain few additives: mashed banana, avocado and tomato, unsweetened natural peanut butter, sunflower or sesame spread, chopped hard-boiled egg, cream cheese, cottage cheese, parsley and natural yoghurt, and sugar-free jam, are all popular. It is important to make the sandwiches look appealing. Younger children like to be able to see what they are eating, so for them the sandwiches should be left open.

Children need no persuading to eat sweet foods. Refined sugar is not nutritious and in the long-term is harmful to health. A small quantity, however, taken occasionally as part of an excellent wholefood diet, probably does little harm. It is not a good idea to insist that the child never eats any food containing sugar, otherwise he may learn to crave it or feel deprived of something his friends all seem to have.

Biscuits may be made at home using wholemeal flour, dried fruit, nuts, butter and a little sugar, honey or concentrated apple juice if necessary. When buying from health-food shops, the labels should be read carefully, and those which contain the least sugar chosen. Ingredients are listed in order by weight, so if sugar is the first or second on the list, they are best avoided. Honey, molasses, glucose, dextrose, sucrose, fructose and malt are all forms of sugar and may appear on the list of ingredients. One should check that the flour used is wholemeal and that there are no artificial additives.

Tiny fairy cakes in miniature paper cases can be made. A favourite recipe is made more nutritious by substituting wholemeal flour for white flour. The amount of sugar in the recipe may be reduced by using raisins, currants or carob powder (a nutritious, naturally sweet, caffeine-free chocolate substitute) instead. The cakes should not be iced.

Dried fruit, carrot or celery sticks, unsalted nuts, pumpkin or sunflower seeds may be put on the table in place of sweets for older children. Children under two should not be allowed nuts or seeds as there is a danger that they might inhale them.

Commercial jelly is better avoided. It contains little but gelatine (a poor-quality protein), sugar, preservative, flavouring and artificial colour. Home-made jelly may be made with unsweetened fruit juices and vegetable jelling compound (from health-food shops). Ice cream is very popular, but many cheap commercial brands are highly processed and lacking in nutrients. If ice cream must be served, then it should be made at home, or a brand chosen which specifies milk or cream as its principal ingredient and contains no additives other than sugar. Alternatively, ice lollies may be made by freezing diluted, unsweetened fruit juice, or fresh fruit mixed with unsweetened natural yoghurt, in lolly moulds. Bananas cut in half and frozen on sticks are also very popular.

Savoury foods, especially crisps, rings, etc., appeal to all ages. They contain a lot of salt, fat and often chemical additives. None of these is conducive to health, especially salt, which has been linked with the development of high blood pressure. If a three- or four-year-old child insists on these types of food at his party, wholegrain alternatives, containing no artificial additives and far less salt and fat, can be found at health-food shops and some supermarkets. Furthermore, unsalted potato crisps are now available. Cheese biscuits containing no added salt are easily made at home.

Sausages, unless they are home made, should rarely, if ever, be given to children. They contain little meat (often of dubious origin), and are high in refined cereals, animal fat and preservatives such as sulphur dioxide or nitrite. Many varieties also contain artificial colour. Savoury alternatives are Cheddar cheese cubes, or little minced meat-balls on cocktail sticks.

It is best to bake the birthday cake at home, going for quality rather than quantity, since children are often too full up to eat it by the time it appears. A suitable recipe should be found, the quantity of sugar reduced and wholemeal flour substituted for white. It may be filled with sugar-free jam if desired. Fresh or dried fruit and a light covering of cream may be used for decoration instead of icing.

Milk or natural fruit juices should replace canned or bottled fizzy drinks and commercial concentrated fruit drinks, which have no place in a child's diet. They contain only a very small percentage of juice, if any, and a lot of sugar, colour and preservative. Cola drinks are particularly harmful, as they contain the stimulant caffeine, which is also present in cocoa, coffee and tea. Caffeine is a drug and children can become addicted to it. It causes sleeplessness and inhibits the absorption of iron. It is a diuretic (a substance which increases the flow of urine from the kidneys), resulting in the loss from the body of B vitamins as well as vitamin C and some minerals. When suddenly deprived of caffeine, a child used to consuming large quantities of it will have withdrawal symptoms, which include headaches, irritability and tiredness.

Artificially sweetened low-calorie drinks are often bought by mothers because they are cheaper than fruit drinks containing sugar. They are essentially solutions of chemicals, however, and until the harmlessness of artificial sweeteners has been proved they should not be given to children.

Here is a check-list for a child's party tea.

| *Conventional party fare* | *Alternative party fare* |
|---|---|
| White bread sandwiches | Wholemeal bread sandwiches |
| Jam | Sugar-free jam |
| Commercial jelly | Home-made jelly* |
| Marmite | Low-salt yeast extract |
| Processed cheese | Cottage or cream cheese |
| Sweetened, commercial peanut butter | Natural peanut butter, sunflower or sesame spread |
| Sweet biscuits | Cheese biscuits* or unsweetened biscuits* |
| Cheap non-dairy ice cream | Home-made ice cream* or ice lollies* |
| Salted crisps | Unsalted crisps |
| Sausages | Meat-balls, cheese cubes |
| Cola, lemonade, squash, Ribena, fruit drinks | Milk, natural fruit juices |
| Chocolate | Carob |

* See recipe section.

## RESTAURANT VISITS

Taking a pre-school child to a restaurant needs a certain amount of planning, if one wants a nutritious meal. The occasional consumption of highly processed foods is unlikely to have a permanent effect on a child's health, but by permitting a child to eat junk foods – even once – he will in all likelihood be hankering for 'those chips' or 'that jelly' long after the event.

The first thing to do when deciding where to go, is to rule out unsuitable restaurants. The least 'healthy' establishments are usually those that serve fast food. Hamburgers, thick milk shakes, chips, southern fried chicken, baked beans and apple pie are not to be recommended for children – despite what persuasive advertising would have one believe. More than 50 per cent of the total energy of these meals comes from fat. They contain a lot of sugar, salt and additives, and are low in fibre.

Restaurants not specifically catering for children, in that they do not provide high chairs or offer children's meals on the menu, often welcome them. When choosing a restaurant, it is wise to select one which is not so smart that the staff will get upset when the child drops food on the floor. Restaurants run by the family-minded Greeks or Italians are a good choice, and turn a blind eye to breast-feeding as long as the mother is discreet. A good method is for her to tuck a napkin into the top of her shirt or jumper and cover the baby's head with it!

Greek restaurants serve very nutritious food. Children should not be given charcoal-grilled meat or fish, however, nor *taramasalata* – an appetizer made from smoked cod's roe, which often contains nitrites and colouring. In Italian restaurants, a plate of pasta with a meat, tomato or cheese sauce can always be served to a child as a main course, and it is sure to keep him busy while the adults are eating. Wholewheat pasta is unlikely to be found on the menu, however.

In English and international restaurants, children can usually be given half portions. Some plain, roast or grilled meat or fish with vegetables is suitable. Sausages, fish-fingers and desserts – other than fruit salad, cheese, etc. – are best avoided. Highly spiced Indian food is not suitable for very young children; nor is most Chinese restaurant food, because it is usually seasoned with monosodium glutamate. The best choice for those not wanting to digress from a wholefood diet is a vegetarian restaurant. Not all of these serve wholegrain dishes, so the meal should be chosen carefully. The restaurants are often self-service and usually serve half portions. Restaurants almost always serve fruit juice. No other drink, other than milk or water, should ever be permitted.

If the child is under a year old, it is advisable to bring a prepared meal from home which he can be given in the restaurant. The staff are unlikely to object if the baby sits in his pushchair while being fed, but may make a small charge if he sits at the table.

## TRAVEL

Travelling with children can be a pleasure or a nightmare, depending on how much preparation has been made for the trip. Taking the right food goes a long way towards making the trip more enjoyable.

Young babies who are totally breast-fed can go anywhere with their mothers without having to have any special arrangements made for them. If the baby is bottle-fed, a made-up bottle of baby milk, a thermos of boiling water and a jug for heating the milk bottle will be needed. Baby milk should never be kept hot in a thermos as it becomes a good breeding ground for bacteria which can cause gastroenteritis. If travelling abroad with a baby, sufficient formula should be taken, as it is unlikely that the same brand will be available abroad.

It is unwise to let young children eat the meals provided on aeroplanes or trains, because of the risk of food poisoning. Jars or cans of commercial baby food are not necessary for short journeys, however, since there are many foods suitable for babies and young children which can be served cold, are easy to prepare and are very nutritious. Sandwiches – the original fast food – make a good meal when made with wholemeal bread and a nutritious filling. Popular fillings include Cheddar cheese, cream cheese and parsley, avocado, egg mayonnaise and cress, unsweetened natural peanut butter or chicken mayonnaise and tomato. Sandwiches can be made the night before, wrapped in plastic film and put in the refrigerator overnight.

Fruit – apples, pears, bananas, etc. – travels well and so does yoghurt (plus spoon). Miniature cartons of pure unsweetened fruit juice complete with straw, are easily transported. Many juices (often called fruit drinks) are sweetened and should be avoided.

Transportable snacks include raisins (in vegetable oil or without oil), unsalted, broken nuts and seeds, wholegrain muesli bars, fruit bars or plain biscuits for older children, and unsalted puffed rice cakes or home-made rusks for babies. Extra food should be prepared in case of delays; one is unlikely to find suitable foods *en route*.

A self-catering holiday is the best idea for those families who wish to keep to a wholefood diet while abroad. Locally produced fresh meat, fish, vegetables and fruit may be purchased and cooked for the child as if at home. Salads should not be given to children as they are often contaminated and all fruit should be peeled. Wholemeal bread and wholegrain cereals may not be easy to find, but pulses are widely available. Fresh pasteurized milk is not always stocked, especially in hot countries. Longlife milk and natural yoghurt may be given instead. Unlike most shops in Britain, many small shops on the Continent have no qualms about selling food which has passed the 'sell by' date, and datemarks should always be checked. It is advisable to buy bottled water for children even if the locals say the tap water is drinkable.

When staying in a hotel, simple foods should be selected from the menu and the child's meat or fish should be well cooked, preferably without seasoning. As a precaution, in this instance, babies who are particularly vulnerable to gastroenteritis should be given commercial baby food, as hotel food and utensils are often contaminated with food-poisoning organisms.

## PICNICS

Picnics can be a lot of fun and do not necessarily require a great deal of preparation. Foods to avoid include synthetic fruit drinks, cola drinks, tea, coffee, alcohol, sweetened commercial yoghurts and desserts, refined bakery products, crisps, most yeast and meat extracts, sweets, chocolates, commercial ice lollies and ice creams, smoked or cured meats or fish (bacon, ham, smoked mackerel, etc.) and barbecued food unless foil wrapped (it is very carcinogenic).

Foods which can be included on a picnic are any fresh meat or fish, fruit, vegetables, wholemeal breads, unsalted seeds (pumpkin, sunflower and sesame), unsalted nuts (hazelnuts, walnuts, peanuts, etc.), dried fruit (unsulphured apricots, raisins in vegetable oil, bananas, etc.), low-sugar muesli bars, fruit bars or biscuits (from health-food shops), salt-free puffed rice cakes, wholegrain crispbread (Ryvita), unprocessed cheese, eggs, natural nut butters (not supermarket brands as they are often hydrogenated and sweetened), unsweetened diluted fruit juices, milk, carob bars (chocolate substitute) and pure juice ice lollies.

If the picnic is to take place when the weather is uncertain, it is a good idea to include hot food. Home-made vegetable and bean soup is very warming. It may be transported in a thermos flask and served in plastic cups. More substantial picnic food may include a cold roast chicken, which can be divided up and eaten with fingers, cold meat-balls, cold fish-balls (made with chopped white fish, onions, egg and breadcrumbs), hard-boiled eggs and cheese cubes.

Vegetables such as raw carrots, cucumber, tomatoes, radishes, cooked new potatoes, cooked chick peas, etc., can be prepared in advance and transported in a plastic sandwich box to accompany meat, fish or eggs. Good picnic fruits are those fruits that do not make a lot of mess when eaten, especially if the picnic is to be eaten in the car. Apples, pears and bananas are all suitable. Oranges, plums and other soft fruits are not ideal for picnics. Small hands and faces get very sticky, and so do clothes.

Sandwiches are perhaps the most convenient picnic food. The fillings should be kept simple, remembering that the under-fives are a pretty conservative bunch. The point to keep in mind about preparing wholefood picnics – as with other meals – is to make the same choice of foods available for children and adults alike. The minute children see crisps, fizzy drinks, etc., they are likely to demand these junk foods in preference to their own nutritious food.

## VISITING GRANDPARENTS

Visiting relatives, such as grandparents, invariably means a departure from a wholefood diet. Many of the older generation are unaware that sugar, white bread, fizzy drinks, etc., are bad for health. They frequently declare that they eat these foods and are still in good shape, and even if they do suffer from poor health, the suggestion that this may be caused by what they eat will be regarded with utter ridicule and disbelief. Grandparents like to give treats, and they know that there is nothing children like better than packets of sweets, crisps or chocolates. They love the chance of spoiling their grandchildren, particularly if they do not see them very often. To avoid unnecessary conflict in these situations, the child's dietary habits should be discussed before the planned visit and on subsequent occasions, as often as it takes for it to sink in. Rather than dictating what the child can't eat, suggestions should be made for fun foods that granny can offer. When she sees that her grandchild is very pleased with his muesli bar, raisins, etc., she will see that he is not 'deprived' and be quite happy to go along with the new plan.

Teatime invariably poses problems. As a show of willingness, grandparents may put a plate of raisins or some fruit on the table, in the misguided belief that if the child only eats wholefoods then he will choose to eat the fruit, raisins, etc., and will reject any junk foods offered. With time, however, as they see their grandchild grow up vigorous and attractive, they are likely to come round to the parents' way of thinking.

When visiting other relatives or friends who are unfamiliar with the child's lifestyle, it is probably not worth the hassle of explaining what he is and is not allowed. They should simply be asked not to offer him any sweets, chocolates, etc. If visitors come to the child's home clutching sweets, the parents should try to intercept them before the child notices. They can then be thrown away (or eaten by the parents) when the visitors have left. If the child is given sweets directly, then they should be taken away with the promise that he can have them later. Later on, if the child is old enough to remember, the sweets may have to be 'swapped' for a small toy or some carob-coated raisins, etc.

# DO'S AND DON'TS

An easy reference guide to what a child may eat

|  | Advisable | In moderation | Strictly limited |
|---|---|---|---|
| Meat | Lamb, beef, poultry, veal, pork, game (without lead shot), offal | Lean minced meat, home-made hamburgers | Bacon, ham, spam, sausages, cured tongue, salt beef, corned beef, commercial meat pies, meat paste, luncheon meat, visible fat on meat |
| Fish | All white fish, all fatty fish (except tuna), fresh fish roe |  | Shellfish, smoked fish, smoked fish roe, fish-fingers, processed fishcakes, etc., canned fish |
| Vegetables | All fresh vegetables, salads, dried pulses | Frozen vegetables | Canned vegetables, chips, potato crisps, olives in brine, pickled cucumbers and onions, chutney |
| Fruit | All fresh fruit | Dates, dried fruit free from mineral oil, sugar or sulphur dioxide | Canned fruit |
| Nuts and seeds | Peanuts, hazelnuts, chestnuts, almonds, brazil nuts, walnuts, cashew nuts | Coconut, sunflower, pumpkin and sesame seeds | Salted nuts, dry roasted nuts |

| | Advisable | In moderation | Strictly limited |
|---|---|---|---|
| Cereal food | Wholegrains – wheat, oats, millet, barley, rice, rye, buckwheat – wholemeal flour, porridge oats, Shredded Wheat, Cubs, Puffed Wheat, unsweetened muesli, wholegrain pasta, wholegrain crispbreads, wholemeal bread | Unbleached 85 per cent extraction flour, Weetabix, low-sugar wholegrain cakes and biscuits, muesli bars, etc., brown bread | White flour, white rice, white spaghetti, cakes and biscuits made with white flour, refined breakfast cereals (most brands), white bread, bran |
| Eggs and dairy produce | Eggs (boiled or scrambled), milk, natural unsweetened yoghurt, butter, Cheddar, Cheshire and soft cheeses | Fried eggs, cream, unsweetened pancakes, home-made unsweetened ice cream | Sweetened yoghurts, milk desserts, processed cheeses, cheese spreads, Edam and Gouda cheeses, custard powder, commercial ice cream |
| Fats and oils | Cold-pressed 'virgin' olive oil, cold-pressed polyunsaturated vegetable oils, unsalted butter, fish oils | Refined olive oil and polyunsaturated oils, soft margarine, salted butter, cream | coconut oil, palm oil, hard margarine, shortening, lard, visible meat fat |
| Drinks | Milk, pure unsweetened fruit juices, water, home-made soup | Low-salt vegetable stock cubes | Tea, coffee, cola drinks, flavoured milk, fruit drinks, squashes or syrups, fizzy drinks, canned or packeted soups, stock cubes, etc. |
| Sweets, preserves and spreads | Natural unsweetened peanut butter and other nut spreads, sesame and sunflower spread, yeast pâté, | A low-salt savoury spread, carob powder (cocoa substitute) | Bovril, Oxo, Marmite, honey, jam, chocolate spread, commercial sweetened peanut butter, lemon curd, meat and fish pastes, |

| | Advisable | In moderation | Strictly limited |
|---|---|---|---|
| | sugar-free jams and marmalade, home-made sugar-free ice lollies | | sweets, chocolates, ice lollies, sugar, salt, artificial sweeteners |
| Snacks | Fresh fruit, raw vegetables, salt-free puffed rice cakes, wholegrain crispbreads (Ryvita), unroasted nuts, diluted fresh fruit juice, milk, cheese | Dried fruit (free from mineral oil, sugar or sulphur dioxide), sugar-free carob- or yoghurt-coated dried fruits and nuts, wholegrain snacks, unsalted potato crisps | All junk food, including sweets, chocolates, fruit drinks, cola, refined bakery products, refined salted snacks |

# QUESTIONS AND ANSWERS

*I want to give my baby the best possible start in life but I have to admit I don't eat a very 'healthy' diet myself. How much does the mother's diet affect the nutritional quality of breast milk?*

Even if the mother's diet is inadequate, the supply of milk is usually maintained. Her own store of nutrients is drawn upon and evidence of malnutrition appears in the mother before it does in her child. It is known that severely malnourished mothers in underdeveloped countries manage to feed their babies for three months before extra food is necessary for the normal growth of the baby.

A mother's diet does, however, affect the concentration of some of the nutrients in milk and also the volume of milk produced. It is therefore apparent that a 'healthy' diet is necessary if the baby is to attain optimum health. Furthermore, the baby of a well-nourished mother is less likely to need supplementary bottle-feeding owing to insufficient breast milk.

*I am breast-feeding my baby and want to wean him straight on to a cup without having to switch to bottles first. How long must I carry on breast-feeding?*

Your baby can start to drink water from a trainer beaker or small cup as soon as he begins to eat a mixed diet (from four months). He can progress to diluted cows' milk when he is six months old, but he will not be good enough at drinking from a cup to get all the fluids he needs until he is seven or eight months old, so he will have to be partially breast-fed at least until then.

*I've heard a lot on the TV about the dangers of animal fat and heart
disease. Is it alright for my children to drink whole milk?*

The fat in milk is highly saturated and raises blood cholesterol levels
when taken in the diet. High cholesterol levels in blood are known
to be associated with heart and blood vessel disease, and for these
reasons the amount of saturated fat in a child's diet should be
limited. Milk fat does, however, contain fat-soluble vitamins A, D
and E, and when the fat is removed these are lost from the diet. While
most doctors recommend that adults do not drink whole milk due to
its high fat content, this recommendation is not intended for children below the age of five, who usually obtain a substantial proportion of dietary energy from cows' milk.

*I often invite my son's friends home for tea but some of them refuse
to eat the 'healthy' food I offer them. Should I buy junk food
specially for these occasions?*

No. If your son's friends don't like 'healthy' food that is just
unfortunate. I doubt whether he will receive any fewer invitations
because of it. I am sure that when your son visits other people's
houses he is not specially catered for, and at least you can feel that
you are not contributing to your son's friends' future bad health.

*My daughter attends a nursery school and the children are given a
biscuit and some orange drink mid-morning. Should I let her eat
this junk food?*

Many children are allergic to oranges so it would not seem unusual
for you to send your child to school with a cup of milk or diluted
apple juice and say she can't tolerate oranges. As for the biscuit, as
long as she is getting a wholefood diet at home, one biscuit a day is
not going to do much harm. Of course, if you wish, you could make
your daughter take her own snack to school. This would make her
feel different, however, which no child enjoys. You will have to
accept that until everyone rejects health-destroying refined foods
there will be times when your child will be offered junk food, and
unless you want her to suffer for your beliefs it is wise not to make
an issue of it.

*My son (aged three) won't eat meat but loves fish. Will he become anaemic?*

While it is true that fish in general does not contain as much well-absorbed iron as liver or red meat, it can contribute a significant amount of iron to the diet. Shellfish contains the most iron but is best avoided as it may produce allergies, is frequently the cause of food poisoning, and concentrates toxic metals such as mercury and cadmium. Good sources of iron are fatty fish such as sardines, sprats and herring, whereas white fish is a poor source. Many vegetables are rich in iron but this iron is less well-absorbed than that from animal foods. Soya beans are a particularly valuable source of iron when the diet does not contain meat; they not only contain a lot of iron, but the iron is also fairly well-absorbed.

As long as your son eats a healthy and varied diet which frequently includes fatty fish, soya beans or bean curd he will not become anaemic.

*I go out to work and employ a nanny to look after my children. How can I make sure they are not eating junk food while I am out?*

It is very important that you explain to any potential employee the kind of diet your family eats. If she proves unsympathetic to your views, then you will have to choose someone else who you feel is prepared to cooperate. Plan your children's lunches for the week and check that all the ingredients are on hand before you leave for work. Also make sure that there are no junk foods in the house. That way there is no risk that your children will find them. Children have a way of knowing where you have hidden the chocolate biscuits long after you have forgotten.

*My child is eleven months old and loves olives. Can I let him eat them?*

No. Olives are bottled in brine (salt water) and are therefore very salty. Even though your baby's kidneys are probably mature enough to handle the amount of salt he would get from eating a few olives, a high salt consumption throughout life, and particularly during a crucial period in childhood, is thought to be one of the factors associated with the development of high blood pressure in later life. All very salty foods are therefore best avoided.

*Can I give my child 'live' yoghurt?*

Yes. 'Live' yoghurt is simply yoghurt which contains the live organisms responsible for turning milk into yoghurt. They are not harmful to health, in fact they are thought to be very beneficial. Almost all commercial yoghurt is 'live' unless it has been pasteurized (e.g. some imported Greek yoghurt). Only 'live' yoghurt can be used as a starter to make yoghurt at home.

*My children are used to sprinkling sugar on their breakfast cereals. How do I stop this habit?*

Young children can usually be persuaded to give up something they like by offering them a tempting alternative. In the case of sugar, a few raisins or sultanas or a ripe banana make a good accompaniment to cereal. At the same time, hide or get rid of all the sugar in the house so that your children have very little choice in the matter. With time they will get used to eating unsweetened foods.

*My children like white bread. If they eat bran on their breakfast cereals will this be as good as eating wholemeal bread?*

No. Supplementing white bread with bran cannot be considered to be nutritionally equivalent to wholemeal bread. When flour is refined, not only is the fibre (bran) removed, but also the germ which is rich in vitamins and minerals. Although some of these nutrients are partially replaced by law, white bread is still far less nutritious than wholemeal. Furthermore, whereas wholemeal bread is only permitted to contain one improver (vitamin C), white bread may contain many bleaches and improvers which are potentially harmful to health.

Bran should never be added to the diet of a young child. It contains a substance called phytic acid which during digestion renders essential minerals (like calcium, iron, magnesium and zinc) unavailable for absorption into the bloodstream. This is particularly harmful to children because of their extra need of nutrients for growth, and because the common infections of childhood increase the rate at which these are used up. Wholemeal bread contains relatively little phytic acid as it is partially degraded by yeast fermentation.

*A lot of health-food products seem to contain honey rather than sugar. Is honey good for you?*

No. Honey is promoted as being a healthy alternative to sugar, which is convenient for manufacturers of wholefood snacks such as muesli bars, biscuits, etc., who would have difficulty selling their products if they were totally unsweetened.

The public sees honey as a healthy food and is eating it in preference to and in addition to jams, syrups and treacle, which are suffering a drop in sales. The sad truth is, however, that honey consists of about 75 per cent sugars and the rest is almost all water, with only traces of other nutrients. It may therefore be considered to be just as harmful to health as sugar.

The only 'advantages' honey has over sugar is that since it is sweeter than sugar, less need be used, and for the same sweetness, honey contains fewer calories.

*My son is two years old and it is inevitable that, sooner or later, he will be introduced to junk foods through his friends and school. Is there any point, therefore, in bringing him up on a wholefood diet during the few years when I can control what he eats and drinks?*

Yes. The eating habits a child acquires during the formative years usually remain with him throughout life. You will find that as your son gets older and has the opportunity to select foods for himself, he will, if given the choice, choose wholefoods in preference to refined foods, even though he might have the occasional lapse and eat sweets, chocolates, etc.

Even if a child were to abandon a wholefood diet at the age of five, the benefits he has attained in terms of superior health and physical development in the years of rapid growth will stand him in good stead for the rest of his life. No parent should willingly pass up the opportunity of giving their child the best possible start.

*I have a weight problem, and am worried that my son (aged nine months) will also have one, so I am weaning him on to a non-fattening diet consisting mainly of skimmed milk, fruit and vegetables. Will it work?*

On this regime, your son is likely to be underweight, and almost certainly lacking in many essential nutrients necessary for optimum health. An adult, health-farm-type diet is totally un-suitable for babies, who need full-fat milk and plenty of energy-rich foods.

As long as your son eats an unrefined diet, then he will thrive without being obese. The diet should contain some food from each of the following groups: carbohydrates (brown rice, wholemeal bread), proteins (meat, fish) and fats (butter, vegetable oils), sup-plemented with fresh fruit and vegetables. Sugar and other refined carbohydrates (white flour products) should be avoided.

*skim*

# RECIPES

## Rice Cereal

Suitable for children over 4 months

1 tablespoon ground brown rice or
  brown rice flour

100 ml (3 ½ fl oz) water

Put the rice in a small saucepan. Mix it to a smooth paste with some
of the water. Blend in the rest of the water and simmer over a low
heat for 5 minutes, stirring constantly. Breast milk or formula may
be added after cooking.

## Muesli

Suitable for children over 6 months

Base
flaked cereal grains (oats, wheat,
  rye, millet)
toasted barley grains
unsulphured* dried fruit (raisins,
  sultanas, apricots, dates)
chopped or flaked nuts (almonds,
  hazelnuts)

To serve
milk
yoghurt
fresh fruit (blackberries, grated
  apple, plum, peach)

Add two parts grains (principally oat flakes), to one part chopped
fruit and nuts. For a child under two years old, process in a food
processor or electric liquidizer. Store in an airtight container.
Muesli may be soaked overnight to make it more digestible. Serve a
small amount of muesli with milk, yoghurt or water and top with a
generous amount of fresh fruit. Only prepare a small quantity of
muesli at one time as it goes rancid quite quickly.

  * See sulphur dioxide, p. 68.

## Wholemeal Bread

Suitable for children over 6 months

750 g (half a bag, 26 oz) of organic
  stone-ground flour
1 sachet Easy Blend Dried Yeast
  (equivalent to 15 g (½ oz)
  ordinary dried yeast or 25 g (1 oz)
  fresh yeast)

1 level teaspoon sea salt
1 dessertspoon cold-pressed
  vegetable oil

Warm a large mixing bowl. Place the flour and the yeast (available from large supermarkets) in the bowl, and stir with a wooden spoon. Heat 500 ml (18 fl oz) water to about 43°C (110°F) and add the salt. Stir until it dissolves. Add the oil to the flour and pour on the water, mixing all the time with the wooden spoon. Knead by hand for a couple of minutes (the dough will be quite sticky). Line the base of a large warmed bread tin with some non-stick baking paper and grease the sides. Press the dough into the tin; it should only half fill it. Cover with a clean tea towel and leave in a warm (but not hot) place to rise for at least 45 minutes or until the dough has nearly doubled in size. Remove the cloth and bake at 190°C (375°F, gas mark 5) for 40 minutes. Turn the loaf out of the tin and cool on a wire rack.

## Rusks

Suitable for children over 6 months

wholemeal bread

Cut 1 cm-thick (½ in) slices of wholemeal bread, remove the crusts and divide into fingers 2 cm (1 in) wide. Bake in a cool oven (150°C, 300°F, gas mark 2) for 20 minutes until firm outside but moist in the centre.

## Beef Broth

Suitable for children over 4 months
serves 6

beef marrow bones
1 oxtail (cut up)
1 onion

3 carrots
1 leek
1 turnip or swede

Wash the bones and oxtail, place in a large saucepan and just cover with water. Bring it to the boil and remove any scum. Prepare the vegetables and add them to the broth. Simmer for 2½ hours, cool and refrigerate overnight. The next day remove the fat and cook for 30 minutes. Serve some meat and vegetables with the broth.

## Grilled Cod
Suitable for children over 4 months

small piece of fresh or frozen cod
   fillet or other white fish
½ teaspoon oil

Wash the fish and place it in a small ovenproof dish, or on a piece of aluminium foil in the grill pan. Brush with a little oil. Grill for about 10 minutes (frozen fish will require longer) without turning, or until the flesh separates into flakes when tested with a fork.

## Beef and Vegetable Hotpot
Suitable for children over 6 months
serves 4

250 g (9 oz) stewing steak
1 dessertspoon wholemeal flour
1 dessertspoon olive oil
1 small onion
1 small turnip or parsnip
1 large carrot
1 broccoli stalk
1 large tomato
½ teaspoon mixed dried herbs or
   some fresh herbs

Wash the meat and dry on kitchen paper. Trim off all visible fat and cut into cubes. Coat the meat with the flour. Heat the oil in a casserole until hot but not smoking. Sear the meat in the hot fat and add the onion chopped finely. Fry the meat and onion for 3 minutes, stirring constantly.

Peel the turnip and carrot, wash the broccoli stalk and tomato and cut them into pieces. Add the vegetables and the herbs to the stew and blend in 100 ml (3½ fl oz) water. Simmer for 1 hour or until the meat is very tender.

## Chopped Liver
Suitable for children over 6 months

1 large onion
1 dessertspoon melted chicken fat
  or butter

125 g (4½ oz) chicken liver
125 g (4½ oz) thinly sliced ox liver

Slice the onion thinly and fry it in the chicken fat over a low heat until soft. Wash the liver, removing any green bits, and pat it dry on kitchen paper. Add the liver to the onions and fry slowly, turning occasionally until the livers are cooked all the way through. Process using a food processor or blender. Refrigerate and serve on wholemeal bread.

## Frittata
Suitable for children over 6 months
makes 4 *frittatas*

1 egg (size 2 or 3)
1 tablespoon milk
2 tablespoons wholemeal flour

6 tablespoons diced cooked mixed
  vegetables
1 tablespoon olive oil

Beat the egg with the milk and blend in the flour. Stir in the cooked vegetables, e.g. mushrooms, green beans, carrots, courgettes, tomatoes, etc. Heat the oil in a frying pan. Drop tablespoonfuls of the mixture into the oil and flatten slightly. Reduce the heat and fry for 2 minutes each side, or until they are light brown.

## Herring Roes
Suitable for children over 6 months
serves 1

4 soft herring roes

1 teaspoon butter

Wash the roes and pat them dry with kitchen paper. Melt the butter in a small frying pan. When the butter begins to bubble, place the roes in the pan. Sauté for a couple of minutes on each side over a low heat. Serve on wholemeal bread and butter.

## Bean Curd, Broccoli, Swede and Parsley Sauce

Suitable for children over 6 months
serves 4

½ small swede
2 stalks broccoli
150 ml (5½ fl oz) water or salt-free
  stock
1 piece bean curd (tofu) (available
  from health-food shops)

*Sauce*
15 g butter
1 tablespoon wholemeal flour
190 ml (⅓ pt) milk
fresh parsley

Peel the swede and cut it into thick sticks. Wash and cut up the broccoli (everything may be eaten). Bring the water or stock to the boil. Add the swede, simmer for 10 minutes, then add the broccoli and lay the bean curd on top of the vegetables so that it steams. Simmer for a further 10 minutes.

While the vegetables are cooking, melt the butter in a small saucepan, stir in the flour, and cook for 1 minute, then work in the milk a little at a time to avoid lumps. Simmer for 3 minutes stirring continuously. Wash some fresh parsley, chop it finely and add it to the sauce just before serving. Serve the bean curd and vegetables and top with some sauce.

## Cheesy Baked Potato

Suitable for children over 6 months
serves 1

1 baking potato
1 teaspoon butter

1 tablespoon grated Cheddar or
  Cheshire cheese

Scrub the potato thoroughly, so that all the dirt is removed. Bake it in a hot oven (for about 1½ hours) until it is tender when tested with a fork. Cut it open lengthways and remove the inside with a spoon, taking care to leave the skin intact. Mash the potato with the butter and grated cheese and pile the filling back into the potato skin, leaving a little grated cheese for the top. For special occasions, cream cheese or soured cream may be substituted for the butter and cheese. Put the potato under the grill to brown the top, and serve. Potatoes cooked the previous day can be used for this recipe. In this case, bake the filled potatoes for 20 minutes prior to serving.

## Scrambled Egg

Suitable for children over 6 months

serves 1

1 egg
1 tablespoon milk

1 teaspoon butter

Beat the egg with the milk. Melt the butter in a pan. When the butter is hot, add the egg mixture, stirring all the time with a wooden spoon. Cook for less than 1 minute until the egg begins to solidify.

## Vegetable Bake

Suitable for children over 6 months

serves 4

1 egg
115 ml (4 fl oz) milk

6 tablespoons cooked diced
    vegetables
40 g (1½ oz) grated Cheddar cheese

Beat the egg with the milk and stir in the vegetables. Pour into a small ovenproof dish. Sprinkle the cheese on top. Bake at 200°C (400°F, gas mark 6) for 15 minutes or until the egg mixture is just set.

## Cottage Pie

Suitable for children over 6 months

serves 4

1 large tomato
100 g (3½ oz) cooked roast beef
    (not more than 1 day old)
1 carrot
½ teaspoon mixed dried herbs

50 ml (scant 2 fl oz) water or
    salt-free stock
1 tablespoon flour
1 large potato
milk

Skin the tomato after plunging it into boiling water for 1 minute. Finely chop the beef and put it into a saucepan with the roughly chopped, scrubbed or peeled carrot, the chopped tomato, the herbs and the water or stock. Bring to the boil and simmer gently for 25 minutes. Mix the flour with a little water, then stir it into the meat. Simmer for a further 5 minutes.

While the meat is cooking, peel the potato, cut it into pieces and plunge it into boiling water. When it is soft, drain off the water and mash the potato with enough milk to give a soft consistency. Spoon the meat and sauce into a dish, cover it with the mashed potato and grill under a hot grill for a few minutes until the top begins to brown.

## Spaghetti Bolognese

Suitable for children over 6 months
serves 4

*Sauce*

½ small onion
1 teaspoon olive oil
100 g (3½ oz) minced steak or
  lean mince
1 dessertspoon wholewheat flour
2 tomatoes

1 carrot
piece of broccoli or 4 mushrooms
  (optional)
100 ml (3½ fl oz) water or salt-free
  stock
100 g (3½ oz) wholewheat spaghetti

Chop the onion finely. Heat the oil and fry the onion until it begins to soften and brown. Stir in the meat and brown it. Sprinkle on the flour and press it into the meat with the back of a wooden spoon. Skin the tomatoes after plunging them in boiling water for 1 minute, chop them and add them to the meat with the finely diced carrot and other vegetables, and the water or stock. Stir, and leave the sauce to simmer for 30 minutes. While the sauce is cooking, boil the spaghetti in 300 ml (11 fl oz) water for 10–12 minutes. Drain, and serve with the sauce.

## Barley and Millet Pilaff

Suitable for children over 6 months
serves 2–4

1 tablespoon pot barley
1 tablespoon millet
200 ml (7 fl oz) water or salt-free
  stock
1 carrot

¼ swede
1 leek

grated cheese

Wash the barley and millet by swirling them in cold water, then draining. Put the barley into a saucepan with the water or stock. Bring to the boil and leave to simmer for 15 minutes. Peel the carrot and swede, dice them and add them to the barley with the millet. After 15 minutes add the washed and finely sliced leek. Cook for a further 10 minutes or until the barley is soft. More water should be added if the pilaff dries out. Serve with a little grated cheese (e.g. Cheddar or Cheshire).

## Meat-Balls

Suitable for children over 6 months
makes 12 meat-balls

1 egg
1 tablespoon wholemeal flour
250 g (9 oz) minced steak or best
  mince

1 teaspoon olive oil
2 tomatoes

Beat the egg and stir in the flour. Blend in the meat and roll the mixture into small meat-balls. Heat the oil in a saucepan. Sear the meat on all sides, then add the coarsely chopped tomatoes and 100 ml (3½ fl oz) water. Simmer for 30 minutes.

## Boiled Chicken and Vegetable Rice

Suitable for children over 6 months
serves 4

1 chicken quarter
1 stalk broccoli
1 small onion
1 small carrot

1 parsnip
1 dessertspoon olive oil
4 tablespoons brown rice

Wash the chicken and broccoli. Peel the onion and scrub or peel the carrot and the parsnip. Heat the oil in a saucepan and fry the finely chopped onion over a moderate heat for a few minutes until it softens, stirring to prevent burning. Add the carefully washed rice, stir and cover with 150 ml (5½ fl oz) water. Place the chicken on top of the rice and surround with the diced vegetables. None of the broccoli need be discarded; the stalk, leaves and head can all be eaten. Bring to the boil and simmer without stirring for 20 minutes. Turn the chicken over and cook for a further 25 minutes or until the rice and chicken are cooked. Add a little more water if necessary.

## Vegetable and Bean Hotpot with Cheese Sauce

Suitable for children over 1 year
serves 4

1 potato
2 carrots
1 tomato
leaf greens (2 or 3 large leaves)
water or salt-free stock (about 200 ml, 7 fl oz)
2 tablespoons cooked borlotti or black-eye beans

Sauce
20 g (¾ oz) butter
1 tablespoon wholemeal flour
190 ml (⅓ pt) milk
50 g (scant 2 oz Cheddar or Cheshire)

Scrub the potato and carrots. Wash the tomato and greens. Bring the water or stock to the boil. Cut up the potato and carrots and plunge them into the boiling water, making sure that the vegetables are not totally submerged; if there is too much water, then discard some. When the potato and carrots are nearly cooked, add the sliced tomato, coarsely shredded greens and the cooked beans. Simmer for a further 5 minutes.

While the vegetables are cooking, prepare the sauce. Melt the butter, stir in the flour, and cook for 1 minute, then blend in the milk over a low heat. Allow the sauce to cook for 3 minutes. Remove from the heat and stir in the grated cheese. Serve the vegetables topped with the sauce.

## Mixed Salad

Suitable for children over 1 year
serves 4

2 very fresh spinach leaves
1 carrot

1 tablespoon bean sprouts

Wash the spinach carefully. Scrub or peel the carrot and rinse the sprouts. Shred the spinach, finely grate the carrot and mix with the sprouts. Serve with a little salad dressing (see next recipe).

## Salad Dressing

Suitable for children over 1 year
serves 4

1 tablespoon cold-pressed polyunsaturated vegetable oil (safflower, sunflower, corn, etc.)

½ teaspoon lemon juice
1 teaspoon natural unsweetened yoghurt

Mix the oil with the lemon juice in a cup. Blend in the yoghurt.

## Baked Beans

Suitable for children over 1 year

250 g (9 oz) dried haricot beans
500 g (18 oz) fresh tomatoes
1 tablespoon olive oil

½ clove garlic
1 teaspoon fresh or ½ teaspoon dried basil or mixed herbs

Wash and drain the beans. Soak them in 3 parts water overnight. Drain, place them in a saucepan, and cover generously with fresh water. Boil them for 10 minutes, then simmer for 1–1½ hours until very tender. Drain and reserve the cooking liquid.

Remove the skins from the tomatoes after plunging them in boiling water for 1 minute. Heat the oil in a casserole dish, crush the garlic and fry it in the oil for 1 minute. Add the herbs and the tomatoes roughly chopped. Simmer for 5–10 minutes until the tomatoes are soft. Stir in the beans and 100 ml (3½ fl oz) of the cooking liquid. Bake in a moderate oven (180°C, 350°F, gas mark 4) for about 1 hour.

## Savoury Millet

Suitable for children over 1 year
serves 2

½ onion
1 teaspoon butter
4 small mushrooms
50 ml (scant 2 fl oz) water or salt-free stock

⅛ teaspoon Natex low-salt yeast extract
3 tablespoons cooked millet
1 dessertspoon unsalted hazelnuts or walnuts

Chop the onion finely and fry it slowly in the butter until it is very soft. Wash the mushrooms, slice them and add them to the onion. Stir in the water or stock, the yeast extract and the cooked millet (see Whole Grains, p. 186). Blend all the ingredients and continue cooking until the millet is hot. Serve and top with the crushed nuts.

## Pizza Toast

Suitable for children over 1 year

serves 2

2 slices wholemeal bread
1 ripe tomato

25 g (1 oz) hard cheese
2 mushrooms

Lightly toast the bread. Skin the tomato after plunging it in boiling water for 1 minute. Chop the tomato finely and spread it on the toast. Slice the cheese thinly or grate it. Layer it on top of the tomato. Wash the mushrooms, slice them and place on top of the cheese. Grill until the cheese begins to bubble.

## Grilled Herring

Suitable for children over 1 year

serves 2

1 small herring

Ask the fishmonger to open up the herring like a kipper, clean it, and remove the centre bone and head. At home, rinse and dry it. Lay it on a baking tray, skin side up, and cook it under a hot grill. After 10 minutes, turn it over and pour off any fat which has come out of the fish. Grill for a further 10 minutes or until the bones become brittle. By cooking the fish for this length of time, the smaller bones may safely be eaten.

## Vegetable Stew

Suitable for children over 1 year

serves 4

2 tablespoons wholewheat grains
1 piece cauliflower
1 potato
1 carrot

8 Brussels sprouts
250 ml (9 fl oz) water or salt-free
 stock
grated cheese

Wash the wheat grains thoroughly. Wash the cauliflower and divide into florets. Scrub the potato and carrot, and remove the outer leaves and the base from the sprouts. Put the wheat and water or stock into a saucepan and bring it to the boil. Simmer for 25 minutes, then add the cut-up potato and carrot. After a further 10 minutes lay the sprouts and cauliflower florets on top. Cook for 15 minutes longer. Serve with grated cheese.

## Barley and Bean Casserole

Suitable for children over 1 year
serves 4

4 tablespoons pot barley
350 ml (12 fl oz) water or salt-free stock
½ swede

1 leek
2 tablespoons cooked pulses

grated cheese

Wash the barley by swirling it in several changes of cold water. Drain it, then place it in a saucepan with the water or stock. Bring it to the boil and simmer for 10 minutes. Peel the swede, dice it and lay it on top of the barley. Simmer for a further 10 minutes. Finally add the washed sliced leek, taking care to remove all the dirt, then the pulses and simmer for another 20 minutes. Serve with a little grated cheese.

## Spaghetti with Vegetable Sauce

Suitable for children over 1 year
serves 4

*Sauce*
1 small onion
1 tablespoon olive oil
1 carrot
1 courgette
1 tablespoon wholewheat flour
2 tomatoes

1 tablespoon cooked pulses
100 ml (3½ fl oz) water or salt-free vegetable stock

100 g (3½ oz) wholewheat spaghetti

Finely chop the onion and fry it in the oil until it begins to brown and soften. Scrub the carrot and wash the courgette, slice them thinly and add them to the onion. Brown them a little, then stir in the flour. Add the coarsely chopped, skinned tomatoes, the pulses and the water or stock, and simmer for 20 minutes, stirring occasionally.

Cook the spaghetti in 300 ml (11 fl oz) boiling water for 10–12 minutes. Drain and serve with the sauce.

## Whole Grains

Wheat, barley, oats, rice, millet and maize are all good to eat, and are popular with young children. Organically grown grain – free from chemical contamination – is best, if it is available. Whole grains have not been processed, so they must be carefully washed before cooking by swirling in two or three changes of cold water, then draining. All grains swell during cooking. Cooked grain may be kept in the refrigerator for 24 hours.

In the following recipes all the cooking water will be absorbed by the grains.

WHEAT:   Use 1 part whole wheat to 2 parts water. Bring to the boil and simmer in a covered saucepan for 50 minutes.

BARLEY:   Use 1 part pot barley to 2 parts water. Bring to the boil and simmer in a covered saucepan for 35 minutes.

OATS:   Use 1 part whole oat groats to 1½ parts water. Bring to the boil and simmer in a covered saucepan for 30 minutes.

RICE:   Use 1 part brown rice to 2 parts water. Bring to the boil and simmer in a covered saucepan, without stirring, for 40 minutes.

MILLET:   Use 1 part millet to 2 parts water. Bring to the boil and simmer in a covered saucepan, without stirring, for 25 minutes.

MAIZE:   Maize may be eaten fresh, as corn cobs. Cook in boiling water for 5–10 minutes, or roast in a hot oven wrapped either in tinfoil or in its own husk.

## Dried Pulses (Beans, Peas, Lentils)

Wash the pulses by swirling them in two or three changes of cold water, then draining. Most pulses (excluding split red lentils, split peas and black-eye beans), must be soaked before cooking. Use 1 part pulses to 3 parts water and soak overnight. Alternatively, bring the pulses to the boil, simmer for 2 minutes, remove from the heat and leave them to soak for 2 hours. Discard the cooking water and cover the pulses generously with fresh water or salt-free stock. Add a dessertspoon of olive oil and 1/2 teaspoon herbs. All pulses must be boiled for 10 minutes at the beginning of the cooking period to destroy certain harmful toxins. Simmer the pulses over a low heat for about 30 minutes for the smallest pulses like aduki or mung, about 1–1½ hours for chick peas, kidney beans or butter beans, and 3–4 hours for soya beans, or until tender. Do not discard the cooking water; it may be used for soup, gravy, etc.

## Fruit Jelly                    Suitable for children over 6 months

vegetable jelling compound       500 ml (18 fl oz) unsweetened pure
                                 fruit juice

Dissolve the jelling compound in some of the juice, according to the manufacturer's instructions. Blend it into the rest of the juice, then bring the juice to the boil, stirring with a wooden spoon. Simmer for 2 minutes. Pour into a mould or individual dishes and leave to set. Fresh fruit (e.g. sliced banana, pear, orange) may be added to the hot jelly.

The following unsweetened juices may be used to make jelly: orange juice, apple juice, red grape juice, pineapple juice.

## Ice Lollies                   Suitable for children over 6 months

FRUIT-JUICE LOLLIES:  unsweetened orange, apple or pineapple juice

Add 1 part juice to 1 part water. Mix and pour into lolly moulds. Freeze.

FRUIT-AND-YOGHURT LOLLIES: natural, unsweetened yoghurt, fresh fruit

Blend 142 g (1 small carton) natural, unsweetened yoghurt with a mashed ripe banana, half a ripe pear, some raspberries, strawberries or blackberries, etc., pour into moulds and freeze.

## Winter Warmer

Suitable for children over 6 months

serves 4

2 eating apples
2 ripe pears

knob of butter
natural, unsweetened yoghurt
raisins

Peel the fruit, quarter and remove the cores. Cook in a saucepan with 1 dessertspoon water and the butter over a low heat until soft. Mash the fruit coarsely and put it into small dishes while still hot. Decorate with yoghurt and chopped raisins.

## Yoghurt

Suitable for children over 6 months

2 teaspoons natural, unsweetened, unpasteurized yoghurt

570 ml (1 pt) UHT milk (full fat)

Add the yoghurt as a starter to UHT (longlife) milk heated to 49°C (120°F). Stir well, or whisk, pour into a spotlessly clean vacuum flask and leave for about 5 hours, or until set, but not solid. Pour the yoghurt into a container, cover and refrigerate immediately. Eat within 1–2 weeks. Two teaspoons of the first batch of yoghurt may be used as starter for the next batch. When the taste begins to deteriorate (after about three batches), some fresh starter will be needed. Either buy a commercial yoghurt or freeze small quantities of the first batch of yoghurt in ice-cube trays, and use one of these as a starter.

The vacuum flask should be sterilized occasionally with a chemical sterilizer used for sterilizing infant feeding bottles. A contaminated vacuum flask will cause the yoghurt to curdle.

## Fresh Fruit Yoghurt

Suitable for children over 6 months

natural, unsweetened yoghurt          fresh fruit

Put the yoghurt in a small dish. Wash or peel some fruit – orange, apple, pear, grapes, melon, plum, raspberries, strawberries, satsuma, banana, etc. Grate or mash the fruit for younger children and babies, cut it into small pieces for older ones. Add it to the yoghurt just before serving.

## Orange Ice Cream

Suitable for children over 6 months*
serves 10

2 large egg whites
140 ml (5 fl oz) double cream

60 ml (2 fl oz) concentrated frozen
orange juice

Whisk the egg whites until they form soft peaks. Whip the cream until thick but not stiff. Blend the concentrated orange juice (this need only be slightly thawed) into the cream. Fold the egg whites gently into the mixture. Freeze until set.

## Apple Snow

Suitable for children over 6 months*
serves 4

2 large sweet eating apples          1 egg white

Peel and core apples. Cut them into thick slices and simmer for about 15 minutes with 1 tablespoon water. Purée and allow to cool. Whisk the egg white until stiff and fold it carefully into the cold apple. Eat within a day.

* Not suitable for babies sensitive to raw egg white.

## Orange Surprise

Suitable for children over 1 year
serves 2

1 orange
2 tablespoons natural, unsweetened
yoghurt

6 grapes

Peel the orange. Slice it into thin rounds. Remove the pips. Put it into two small dishes. Cover the orange slices with a tablespoon of yoghurt. Decorate with grape halves.

## Apple Buns

Suitable for children over 1 year
makes 12 buns

200 g (7 oz) wholemeal self-raising
flour
50 g (scant 2 oz) raisins
50 g (scant 2 oz) desiccated coconut
or chopped dates
2 level teaspoons cinnamon

¼ teaspoon grated nutmeg
2 eating apples
60 g (2 oz) butter
1 egg (size 1 or 2)
milk

Put the flour, washed raisins, coconut or dates, and the spices in a large mixing bowl. Wash, but do not peel the apples and grate them using a coarse grater. Melt the butter and beat the egg. Combine all the ingredients thoroughly to form a stiff mixture. Add a little milk if necessary.

Spoon the mixture into a bun tin and bake at 190°C (375°F, gas mark 5) for 15–20 minutes.

## Strawberry Fool

Suitable for children over 1 year
serves 6

1 egg white (size 1 or 2)
115 ml (4 fl oz) double cream

150 g (5½ oz) strawberries (or
raspberries or blackberries)

Whisk the egg white until it is stiff. Whip the cream until it begins to thicken. Mash the washed berries. Blend the berries with the cream and carefully fold in the egg white. Spoon into small dishes and refrigerate. Eat within 12 hours.

## Fruit Boats

1 large eating apple          6 grapes
1 satsuma or ½ orange

Wash the apple. Cut it lengthways into six equal pieces and remove the core. Peel the satsuma or orange and divide it into segments. Place one segment on each apple boat and spear it and the apple with a cocktail stick. Wash the grapes and remove the pips. Push a grape on to the top of each cocktail stick.

## Hawaiian Cocktail

1 slice fresh pineapple or an orange          1 dessertspoon raisins
1 banana          1 dessertspoon desiccated coconut

Remove the peel and core from the pineapple, and cut it into chunks. Peel and slice the banana. Wash the raisins in hot water. Mix the pineapple, banana and raisins together. Put it into two dishes and decorate with coconut.

## Unsweetened Biscuits

100 g (3½ oz) hazelnuts          50 g (scant 2 oz) raisins
100 g (3½ oz) butter          2 level teaspoons cinnamon
1 egg (size 1 or 2)          200 g (7 oz) wholemeal flour

Process the hazelnuts in a food processor, then the cut-up butter, egg, rinsed raisins, cinnamon and flour. Alternatively, crush the hazelnuts by putting them in a plastic bag and banging it with a rolling pin, then place the crushed nuts in a bowl and add the other ingredients, one at a time. Carefully roll out the dough on a floured board to a thickness of about 6 mm (¼ in). Cut with a biscuit cutter and bake at 190°C (375°F, gas mark 5) for 15–20 minutes until they begin to brown. Cool on a wire rack.

192 • A Good Start

## Cheese Biscuits

Suitable for children over 1 year
makes 25 small biscuits

NOV 87

125 g (4½ oz) wholemeal flour
75 g (2½ oz) grated mature
   Cheddar cheese
50 g (scant 2 oz) butter

1 egg yolk
cayenne pepper
milk or water
raisins

Mix the flour with the cheese, butter, egg yolk and a very small
pinch of cayenne pepper. Beat, process or knead by hand to form a
stiff dough, adding some milk or water if the dough is too dry. Roll
out the dough on a floured board to a thickness of about 3 mm (⅛ in),
and cut it into animal shapes using special biscuit cutters. Use the
raisins to make eyes. Bake for 10–15 minutes at 190°C (375°F, gas
mark 5) until they begin to brown. Cool on a wire rack.

4 oz. FLOUR   for 2 cookie sheets
1½ BUTTER

# WEIGHTS AND MEASURES

The metric/imperial conversions used throughout this book are convenient approximations.

## Weights

| | | |
|---|---|---|
| 1 milligram (mg) | = | 1,000 micrograms (µg) |
| 100 grams (g) | = | 3.53 oz |
| 1 kilogram (kg) | = | 2.20 lb |
| 1 ounce (oz) | = | 28.35 g |
| 1 pound (lb) | = | 453.6 g |

## Fluid measures

| | | |
|---|---|---|
| 100 millilitres (ml) | = | 3.52 fl oz |
| 1 litre (l) | = | 1.76 pt |
| 1 fluid ounce (fl oz) | = | 28.41 ml |
| 1 pint (pt) | = | 568.3 ml |

## Energy

| | | |
|---|---|---|
| 1 kilojoule (kJ) | = | 1,000 joules (J) |
| 1 megajoule (MJ) | = | 239 kcal |
| 1 kilocalorie (kcal) | = | 4.184 kJ |

# BIBLIOGRAPHY

AGRICULTURAL RESEARCH COUNCIL/MEDICAL RESEARCH COUNCIL, *Food and Nutrition Research*, London, HMSO, 1974.

BALLENTINE, R., *Diet and Nutrition: A Holistic Approach*, Honesdale, The Himalayan International Institute, 1978.

BINGHAM, S., *Nutrition: A Consumer's Guide to Good Eating*, London, Corgi Books, 1978.

BIRCHER-BENNER, M., *Children's Diet Book*, Connecticut, Keats Publishing, 1977.

BRITISH SOCIETY FOR POPULATION STUDIES, *Measuring Sociodemographic Change*, London, OPCS, 1985.

CLEAVE, T. L., *The Saccharine Disease*, Bristol, John Wright, 1974.

DAVIDSON, SIR STANLEY, and others, *Human Nutrition and Dietetics*, Edinburgh, Churchill Livingstone, 1979.

DAVIS, ADELLE, *Let's Have Healthy Children*, 3rd ed., London, Allen & Unwin, 1981.

DEPARTMENT OF HEALTH AND SOCIAL SECURITY, *Artificial Feeds for the Young Infant* (Report on Health and Social Subjects, 18), London, HMSO, 1980.

DEPARTMENT OF HEALTH AND SOCIAL SECURITY, *Breast Feeding*, London, HMSO, 1978.

DEPARTMENT OF HEALTH AND SOCIAL SECURITY, *Diet and Cardiovascular Disease* (Report on Health and Social Subjects, 28), London, HMSO, 1984.

DEPARTMENT OF HEALTH AND SOCIAL SECURITY, *Lead and Health: The Report of a DHSS Working Party on Lead in the Environment*, London, HMSO, 1980.

DEPARTMENT OF HEALTH AND SOCIAL SECURITY, *Nutritional Aspects of Bread and Flour* (Report on Health and Social Subjects, 23), London, HMSO, 1981.

DEPARTMENT OF HEALTH AND SOCIAL SECURITY, *Present-day Practice in Infant Feeding: 1980* (Report on Health and Social Subjects, 20), London, HMSO, 1980.

DEPARTMENT OF HEALTH AND SOCIAL SECURITY, *Recommended Daily*

*Amounts of Food Energy and Nutrients for Groups of People in the United Kingdom* (Report on Health and Social Subjects, 15), London, HMSO, 1979.

DEPARTMENT OF HEALTH AND SOCIAL SECURITY, *Vitamin D Deficiency and Osteomalacia* (Topics of Our Time, 1), London, HMSO, 1976.

FOMON, S. J., *Infant Nutrition*, 2nd ed., Philadelphia, W. B. Saunders, 1974.

FOX, B. A., and CAMERON, A. G., *Food Science*, 4th ed., London, Hodder & Stoughton, 1982.

LAPPÉ, F. M., *Diet for a Small Planet*, new ed., New York, Ballantine Books, 1982.

MCLAREN, D. S., and BURMAN, D., *Textbook of Paediatric Nutrition*, 2nd ed., Edinburgh, Churchill Livingstone, 1982.

MINISTRY OF AGRICULTURE, FISHERIES AND FOOD, *Manual of Nutrition*, London, HMSO, 1976.

NACNE, *Proposals for Nutritional Guidelines for Health Education in Britain*, London, Health Education Council, 1983.

PAUL, A. A., and SOUTHGATE, D. A. T., *The Composition of Foods*, London, HMSO, 1978.

PRICE, W. A., *Nutrition and Physical Degeneration: A Comparison of Primitive and Modern Diets and their Effects*, La Mesa, Price-Pottenger Nutrition Foundation, 1970.

STANWAY, A. and P., *Breast is Best*, 2nd ed., London, Pan Books, 1983.

Reference has also been made to articles in various journals, including:

*Science; Lancet; British Medical Journal; British Journal of Preventive and Social Medicine; Nutrition and Food Science; Archives of Disease in Childhood; Proceedings of the Nutrition Society; Journal of the American Medical Association; Nutrition Reviews; British Journal of Nutrition.*

# GENERAL INDEX

and vitamin C, 36, 143
and weaning, 126, **127–8**
deficiency, 17, 77, 124
in eggs, 101
in fish, 102, 170
in molasses, 64
in refined flour, 65
in soya beans, 153
in vegan diet, 151
in vegetables, 154
in vegetarian diet, 170
in whole grains, 65, 152

jam, 108, 147
jellies, 143, 157–8
   home-made, 158
jelling compound, 158
junk foods, 11, 12, 14, **56–7**, 62, 144,
   150, 156, 163, 169, 172
   and eating problems, 147
   and restaurants, 159–60
   and salt consumption, 16
   and vitamins, 16

kelp, 109
kidneys, 21, 31, 121
   and diabetes, 89
   and diuretic foods, 159
   and high blood pressure, 85
   and lead, 76
   and potassium, 46
   and salt consumption, 15–16, 47,
      125, 136
   in infants, 15–16, 125, 136, 170
kitchenware, 90
knock knees, 39
koh-koh, 106, 129
*kombu*, 109

labelling of foods, 69, 98, 104–5,
   109, 137, 162
lactic acid, 60, 61, 69, 71
lactose, 25, 60–61, 120
   and dental caries, 80
   in breast milk, 118
   in cows' milk, 58, 118
   in infant formula milk, 118, 119
La Leche League, 115

lard, 27
laxatives, 29, 87, 127
lead, 19, 51, 64, **76–7**, 92, 122
leaves, starch in, 27
lecithin, 29, 62, 63
lentils, 107–8, 153
linoleic acid, 28
liquidizer, 91
liver, 48, 51, 71
   and cholesterol, 29
   and vitamins, 31, 32, 35–6, 38
   cancer of the, 88
lunch, 146
   menus, 132, 133, 145

MSG (621), monosodium
   glutamate, 18, 46, **70**, 86, 105, 160
macaroni, 66, 129
macrobiotic diet, 40
magnesium, 42, **47–8**, 97, 171
magnesium salts (Epsom salts), 48
main meal, 142, **143**
   menus, 132, 133, 145
maize (Indian corn), **67**, 152
malic acid, 71
malnutrition, 25
malt, 56
malt extract, 67, 80
maltodextrins, 119
maltose, 25, 67, 80, 137
manganese, 42, **52**
maranta, West Indian, 67
margarine, 14, 28, **61–2**, 63
   and vitamins, 31, 38
markets, 98
Marmite, 86, 108, 134
meals, *see* menus
measles, 112, 149
meat
   and fat, 14, 27, 28
   and iron consumption, 48
   and modern urban diet, 53
   and potassium, 45
   and vitamins, 35
   and zinc, 50
   cured, 102, 128, 134; additives in,
      68; and cancer, 69, 88; and salt,
      86

raisins, 58, 71
rashes, 70, 112, 127, 129
raspberries, 87
rationing, 11
raw foods, 53, 54, 144
recipes, 174–92; *see also* separate
   recipe index
refined foods, 12, 21, 46, 53, 79–89,
   146–7, 149
   and babies, 138; *see also*
     commercial baby foods
   and dietary fibre, 15
   and vitamin consumption, 16
   *see also* flour, sugar, etc.
rennet, 60
respiration, 39, 74, 138
restaurants, 159–60
retinol, *see* vitamin A
Ribena, baby, 137
riboflavin (vitamin B2), 32, **33**, 58,
   102, 151
rice, 66
   and weaning, 106, 107, 125, 129,
     152
   cakes, brown, 106
Rice Crispies, 86
rickets, 17, **39–40**, 43, 116, 138
roasting, 97
rusks, 13, 81, 125, 130, 137
rye, 67, 143
Ryvita, 143, 162

SMA, 119
SMA Gold Cap, 119
saccharin, **70**, 88
sago, 27, 67
salad dressing, 144
salads, 161, 146
salmonella, 93, **94**
salt (sodium chloride), 16, 42, 45,
    **46–7**, 53, **85**, 88, 134, 144
   and blood vessel disease, 82
   and high blood pressure, **85**, 170
   and kidneys, 121
   and monosodium glutamate, 70
   and weaning, 125
   as a preservative, 69
   deficiency of, 47

in butter, 60, 102
in cheese, 60, 101
in commercial baby foods, 136
in cured fish, 103
in fruit juices and syrups, 46, 138
in infant formula milk, 118,
   119–20, 122
in junk foods, 109, 146, 156, 158,
   160
in margarine, 61
in olives, 170
in refined breakfast cereals, 108,
   143
in yeast extracts, 109
sandwiches, 161, 163
   fillings, 108–9, 130, 143, 152,
    157, 161, 166
sauces, 148
sausages, 158
   black, 48
scurvy, 17, 30, 37–8
seafood, 18, 50, 51; *see also* fish,
   shellfish, etc.
seaweed products, 109
seborrheoic dermatitis (cradle cap), 35
seeds, 27, 28, 35, 107, 154
   and protein complementarity, 23,
    152
   sprouting, 153
   *see also* cereals and grains, and
    names of individual seeds
selenium, 42
semolina, 66
sesame seeds, 152
shellfish, 19, 76, 78, 103, 128, 170
shopping
   for fresh foods, 98–105
   for health foods, 105–10
Shredded Wheat, 84, 108, 129, 142
sick children, 148, 149–50
skin, 13, 30, 38
sleep disturbances, 76
smoke and smoked foods, 69, 78,
   88, 95
smoking (cigarettes), 82, 114, 115
snacks, 14, 16, 62, **144–6**, 148
   wholefood, 109, 144, 157, 158,
    161, 166, 172

# RECIPE INDEX

## MORE ABOUT PENGUINS, PELICANS, PEREGRINES AND PUFFINS

For further information about books available from Penguins please write to Dept EP, Penguin Books Ltd, Harmondsworth, Middlesex UB7 ODA.

*In the U.S.A.*: For a complete list of books available from Penguins in the United States write to Dept DG, Penguin Books, 299 Murray Hill Parkway, East Rutherford, New Jersey 07073.

*In Canada*: For a complete list of books available from Penguins in Canada write to Penguin Books Canada Ltd, 2801 John Street, Markham, Ontario L3R 1B4.

*In Australia*: For a complete list of books available from Penguins in Australia write to the Marketing Department, Penguin Books Australia Ltd, P.O. Box 257, Ringwood, Victoria 3134.

*In New Zealand*: For a complete list of books available from Penguins in New Zealand write to the Marketing Department, Penguin Books (N.Z.) Ltd, Private Bag, Takapuna, Auckland 9.

*In India*: For a complete list of books available from Penguins in India write to Penguin Overseas Ltd, 706 Eros Apartments, 56 Nehru Place, New Delhi 110019.

*THE PENGUIN HEALTH SERIES*

## THE PENGUIN ENCYCLOPAEDIA OF NUTRITION John Yudkin

This book cuts through all the myths about food and diets to present the real facts clearly and simply. 'Everyone should buy one' – *Nutrition News and Notes*

## THE PRIME OF YOUR LIFE
Dr Miriam Stoppard

The first comprehensive, fully illustrated guide to healthy living for people aged fifty and beyond, by top medical writer and media personality, Dr Miriam Stoppard.

## HOW TO GET OFF DRUGS Ira Mothner and Alan Weitz

This book is a vital contribution towards combating drug addiction in Britain in the eighties. For drug abusers, their families and their friends.

## THE ROYAL CANADIAN AIRFORCE XBX PLAN FOR PHYSICAL FITNESS FOR MEN
*and*
## THE ROYAL CANADIAN AIRFORCE XBX PLAN FOR PHYSICAL FITNESS FOR WOMEN

Get fit and stay fit with minimum fuss and maximum efficiency, using these short, carefully devised exercises.

## PREGNANCY AND CHILDBIRTH
Sheila Kitzinger

A complete and up-to-date guide to physical and emotional preparation for pregnancy – a must for prospective parents.

## ALTERNATIVE MEDICINE Andrew Stanway

Dr Stanway provides an objective and practical guide to thirty-two alternative forms of therapy – from Acupuncture and the Alexander Technique to Macrobiotics and Yoga.

## NATUREBIRTH Danaë Brook

A pioneering work which includes suggestions on diet and health, exercises and many tips on the 'natural' way to prepare for giving birth in a joyful relaxed way.

*OTHER PENGUIN BOOKS ON HEALTH*

## A COMPLETE GUIDE TO THERAPY
Joel Kovel

The options open to anyone seeking psychiatric help are both numerous and confusing. Dr Kovel cuts through the many myths and misunderstandings surrounding today's therapy and explores the pros and cons of various types of therapies.

## PREGNANCY Dr Jonathan Scher and Carol Dix

Containing the most up-to-date information on pregnancy – the effects of stress, sexual intercourse, drugs, diet, late maternity and genetic disorders – this book is an invaluable and reassuring guide for prospective parents.

## YOGA Ernest Wood

'It has been asked whether in yoga there is something for everybody. The answer is "yes" ' Ernest Wood

## DEPRESSION Ross Mitchell

Depression is one of the most common contemporary problems. But what exactly do we mean by the term? In this invaluable book Ross Mitchell looks at depression as a mood, as an experience, as an attitude to life and as an illness.

## VOGUE NATURAL HEALTH AND BEAUTY Bronwen Meredith

Health foods, yoga, spas, recipes, natural remedies and beauty preparations are all included in this superb, fully illustrated guide and companion to the bestselling *Vogue Body and Beauty Book*

## CARE OF THE DYING Richard Lamerton

It is never true that 'nothing more can be done' for the dying. This book shows us how to face death without pain, with humanity, with dignity and in peace.

*OTHER PENGUIN BOOKS ON HEALTH*

## AUDREY EYTON'S F-PLUS Audrey Eyton

'Your short-cut to the most sensational diet of the century' – *Daily Express*

## CARING WELL FOR AN OLDER PERSON Muir Gray and Heather McKenzie

Wide-ranging and practical, with a list of useful addresses and contacts, this book will prove invaluable for anyone professionally concerned with the elderly or with an elderly relative to care for.

## BABY AND CHILD Penelope Leach

A beautifully illustrated and comprehensive handbook on the first five years of life. 'It stands head and shoulders above anything else available at the moment' – Mary Kenny in the *Spectator*

## WOMAN'S EXPERIENCE OF SEX
Sheila Kitzinger

Fully illustrated with photographs and line drawings, this book explores the riches of women's sexuality at every stage of life. 'A book which any mother could confidently pass on to her daughter – and her partner too' – *Sunday Times*

## PROBLEM DRINKING Nick Heather and Ian Robertson

Alcoholism is a terrible scourge, but it can be successfully treated once it is understood to be a socially learned behavioural disorder. This is a very valuable book for sufferers, their families and therapists.

## PREGNANCY AND DIET Rachel Holme

It *is* possible to eat well and healthily when pregnant while avoiding excessive calories; this book, with suggested foods, a sample diet-plan of menus and advice on nutrition, shows how.

*COOKERY IN PENGUINS*

## MEDITERRANEAN FOOD Elizabeth David

Based on a collection of recipes made when the author lived in France, Italy, the Greek Islands and Egypt, this was the first book by Britain's greatest cookery writer.

## THE COMPLETE BARBECUE BOOK
James Marks

Mouth-watering recipes and advice on all aspects of barbecuing make this an ideal and inspired guide to *al fresco* entertainment.

## A BOOK OF LATIN AMERICAN COOKING Elisabeth Lambert Ortiz

Anyone who thinks Latin American food offers nothing but *tacos* and *tortillas* will enjoy the subtle marriages of texture and flavour celebrated in this marvellous guide to one of the world's most colourful *cuisines*.

## QUICK COOK Beryl Downing

For victims of the twentieth century, this book provides some astonishing gourmet meals – all cooked in under thirty minutes.

## JOSCELINE DIMBLEBY'S BOOK OF PUDDINGS, DESSERTS AND SAVOURIES

'Full of the most delicious and novel ideas for every type of pudding' – *Lady*

## CHINESE FOOD Kenneth Lo

A popular step-by-step guide to the whole range of delights offered by Chinese cookery and the fascinating philosophy behind it.

## A NEW BOOK OF MIDDLE EASTERN FOOD Claudia Roden

'It has permanent value' – Paul Levy in the *Literary Review*. 'Beautifully written, interesting and evocative' – Josceline Dimbleby in the *Sunday Telegraph*. This revised and updated edition of *A Book of Middle Eastern Food* contains many new recipes and much more lore and anecdote of the region.

## THE PLEASURE OF VEGETABLES Elizabeth Ayrton

'Every dish in this beautifully written book seems possible to make and gorgeous to eat' – *Good Housekeeping*

## FRENCH PROVINCIAL COOKING Elizabeth David

'One could cook for a lifetime on this book alone' – *Observer*

## JANE GRIGSON'S FRUIT BOOK

Fruit is colourful, refreshing and life-enhancing; this book shows how it can also be absolutely delicious in meringues or compotes, soups or pies.

## A TASTE OF AMERICAN FOOD Clare Walker

Far from being just a junk food culture, American cuisine is the most diverse in the world. Swedish, Jewish, Creole and countless other kinds of food have been adapted to the new environment; this book gives some of the most delicious recipes.

## LEAVES FROM OUR TUSCAN KITCHEN Janet Ross and Michael Waterfield

A revised and updated version of a great cookery classic, this splendid book contains some of the most unusual and tasty vegetable recipes in the world.